CLARK'S

ESSENTIAL GUIDE TO

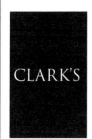

OPERATIONAL MANAGEMENT AND BUSINESS PRACTICE IN MEDICAL IMAGING AND RADIOTHERAPY

This easy-to-understand pocketbook in the highly respected Clark's series of diagnostic imaging texts introduces practitioners and students to the concepts of management, leadership and business planning, and outlines the knowledge and skills required to maintain the daily functioning of a medical imaging and radiotherapy department. Recognising that the transition from clinical radiographer to team lead or manager can be challenging, the book provides a good knowledge of management functions that will assist in this development and enable further progression into operational management roles.

Clark's Essential Guide to Operational Management and Business Practice in Medical Imaging and Radiotherapy takes the systematic approach adopted within books in the Clark's series and is designed to be clear and consistent, introducing the reader to differing concepts of management. All involved in managing imaging delivery and practice, no matter what the area of service, will benefit greatly from this publication.

CLARK'S COMPANION ESSENTIAL GUIDES

Series Editor
A. Stewart Whitley

Clark's Essential PACS, RIS and Imaging Informatics
Alexander Peck

Clark's Essential Physics in Imaging for Radiographers, Second Edition
Ken Holmes, Marcus Elkington, Phil Harris

Clark's Essential Guide to Clinical Ultrasound
Jan Dodgeon, Gill Harrison

Clark's Essential Guide to Mammography
Claire Borrelli, Claire Mercer

Clark's Pocket Handbook for Radiographers, Third Edition
A. Stewart Whitley, Charles Sloane, Gail Jefferson, Ken Holmes, Craig Anderson

Clark's Essential Guide to Mobile and Theatre Imaging
Amanda Martin, Ken Holmes, Andrea Hulme, Helen Fowler

Clark's Essential Guide to Operational Management and Business Practice in Medical Imaging and Radiotherapy
Amanda Martin, Peter Hogg, Philip Webster, Louise Kemp, Lesley Wright

https://www.routledge.com/Clarks-Companion-Essential-Guides/book-series/CRCCLACOMESS

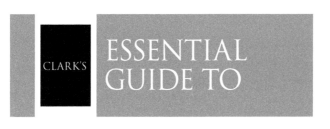

CLARK'S ESSENTIAL GUIDE TO

OPERATIONAL MANAGEMENT AND BUSINESS PRACTICE IN MEDICAL IMAGING AND RADIOTHERAPY

Edited by

Amanda Martin
Radiography Consultant and Lecturer, University of Cumbria, UK

Peter Hogg
Professor Emeritus, University of Salford, UK

Philip Webster
Technical Advisor to Alliance Medical Limited, UK

Louise Kemp
Workforce, Training and Projects Manager, Previous PACS Manager
and Service Lead, UK

Lesley Wright
Healthcare Systems Engineer and Diagnostic Specialist Advisor, UK

With additional contributions from
Jo Cresswell

Series Editor for *Clark's Companion Essential Guides*:

A. Stewart Whitley
Radiology Advisor, UK Radiology Advisory Services, Preston, Lancashire,
UK and Former Director of Professional Practice for the International
Society of Radiographers and Radiological Technologists (ISRRT)

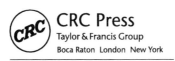

CRC Press
Taylor & Francis Group
Boca Raton London New York

CRC Press is an imprint of the
Taylor & Francis Group, an **informa** business

Designed cover image: iStock™ image number 1319849784. Credit: Andres Victorero

First edition published 2025
by CRC Press
2385 NW Executive Center Drive, Suite 320, Boca Raton, FL 33431

and by CRC Press
4 Park Square, Milton Park, Abingdon, Oxon, OX14 4RN

CRC Press is an imprint of Taylor & Francis Group, LLC

© 2025 selection and editorial matter: Amanda Martin, Peter Hogg, Philip Webster, Louise Kemp and Lesley Wright; individual chapters: the contributors

ISBN: 978-1-032-45302-6 (hbk)
ISBN: 978-1-032-43615-9 (pbk)
ISBN: 978-1-003-38007-8 (ebk)

DOI: 9781003380078

Typeset in Linotype Berling LT Std
by Evolution Design and Digital Ltd (Kent)

CONTENTS

FOREWORD

It has been a delight to witness the development and publication of *Clark's Essential Guide to Operational Management and Business Practice in Medical Imaging and Radiotherapy.*

This latest addition to the Clark's series of pocket and desktop books is a testament to the skills, knowledge and dedication of the authors, who have at heart the desire to share their knowledge and experience with radiographers engaged in this area of expertise.

The success of any organisation is dependent on good leadership and the management skills of those in authority and tasked with delivering a service. This book is aimed at those radiographers who may wish to take up, or have taken up, junior management roles and who are motivated to progress up the management career ladder to further their career in more senior roles.

Patients and users of our services, including commissioners, deserve to know and be assured that those managing diagnostic imaging and radiotherapy services are competent, skilled and knowledgeable of all those aspects and conditions that ensure a safe and effective service and environment.

This book will introduce the reader to differing concepts of management, and outline the knowledge and skills required to maintain the daily functioning of a medical imaging and/or radiotherapy department.

Miss K. C. Clark, I am sure, would welcome this important addition to the *Clark's Companion Essential Guides.*

I am confident that all involved in managing, no matter what the area of service, will benefit greatly from this publication.

A. Stewart Whitley
Series Editor
Former ISRRT Director of Professional Practice &
Radiology Advisor
UK Radiology Advisory Services
Preston, Lancashire, UK

PREFACE

This first edition of *Clark's Essential Guide to Operational Management and Business Practice in Medical Imaging and Radiotherapy* is a comprehensive guide to support practitioners aspiring to be future leaders or managers. Throughout the text, the term 'leader' will be used. This encompasses both management and leadership roles as, while a leader does not necessarily need to manage, a manager does need to lead. The book introduces the philosophies of leadership and the practicalities of operational management and business practices at a level that is easy to understand.

Many purchasers of medical imaging services encourage those providers to demonstrate that their services have been subject to an accreditation process with an appropriate accreditation body. In the UK, this is the UK Accreditation Service, which is responsible for assessing the competence of an organisation against standards developed by the professional bodies associated with that organisation. The Quality Standard for Imaging (QSI) has been developed by the Royal College of Radiologists and the College of Radiographers (available at *www.rcr.ac.uk/our-services/management-service-delivery/quality-standard-for-imaging-qsi/*); it ensures that standards are being met in all aspects of service delivery and patient care. Independent regulators, such as the Care Quality Commission (CQC) in England, the Care Inspectorate in Scotland and Wales and the Regulation and Quality Improvement Authority in Northern Ireland, are likely to look favourably at a service that is accredited, as it demonstrates that key quality standards are being met. The purpose of the independent regulators is to ensure that health and social care services, regardless of the provider, meet the required standards of both quality and safety. They will conduct inspections of services, either planned or unplanned, and measure them against predetermined standards. Depending on the regulator, those standards may include the safety of the environment in which care is being delivered, the procedures in place to respond to complaints, risk and incident management, staffing and the leadership of the organisation.

This book introduces a broad range of topics, many of which can be found in the QSI and/or CQC standards. The purpose is not to deliver detailed text, but to enable the practitioner to familiarise themselves with the principles and language associated with each topic. This can then be further developed as the practitioner progresses down their chosen career path.

Several of these topics are highly specialised and demand competent professionals who know the intricacies of the field. Consequently, in the early stages of creating this book, it became clear that we needed a range of people with the right knowledge to write the chapters. Our author team grew as the book contents started to take shape and additional authors were included as time progressed. The diverse nature of knowledge needed to be a successful leader, as illustrated in the book chapters, necessitated a need for a significant change in the way this Clark's book has been managed – from concept to publication; this change has also driven how contributors have been acknowledged for their work. Until now, Clark's books have been 'authored' books. Here, all the authors worked together to write, and then to take collective responsibility for, the contents. Owing to the diverse nature of the subjects in the chapters of this book, not all authors were able to contribute intellectual input to all chapters. For this reason, this management book is an 'edited' book. Each chapter bears the name(s) of the author(s) who wrote it; for the book overall, the book editors have taken responsibility for ensuring that chapter authors produce the right standard of material, in the right format and style.

Given the ever-changing landscape of health and social care delivery, it is necessary to say that this book has been developed using information and practices that are current at the time of writing. Descriptions of leadership theories will remain the same, but budget management and procurement practice may change, so it is important to make sure that the latest information is being used when applying it to practice.

Amanda Martin
Peter Hogg
Philip Webster
Louise Kemp
Lesley Wright

BIOGRAPHIES

Editors

Dr Amanda Martin has worked in various specialties and roles during her extensive clinical and academic radiography career, including as a Lecturer Practitioner, as a Programme Lead for MSc in Advanced Practice and, for the last 15 years of her career, as a Clinical Manager and a Lead Radiographer. She was among the first radiographers to independently report X-ray images and achieved an MSc in 1999, a Postgraduate Certificate in Learning and Teaching for Higher Education in 2007 and a Professional Doctorate in Health and Social Care in 2011. She was awarded the Fellowship of the College of Radiographers in 2019. During her career, Dr Martin has presented at numerous national and international conferences and had many publications. Since 2022, she has been working as a Radiography Consultant in the UK, supporting education programmes and advising on product development, while still reporting on musculoskeletal images within the NHS. She is an author of multiple Clark's publications.

Professor Peter Hogg's involvement in management and leadership started early. In his mid-20s, Professor Hogg became acting superintendent radiographer in charge of a research institute to cover maternity leave. At 30, he became a master's degree course leader, a role he held for 18 years. In the university sector, he has held several appointments, including Head of Department, Associate Dean (Research), Research Centre Director and Lead for the Diagnostic Imaging Research Programme. Within the radiography profession, across several decades, he has sat on many national and international committees. Examples of these include the *Radiography* journal's editorial board – he was Editor-in-Chief for several years; he was an Associate Editor for the (American) *Journal of Nuclear Medicine Technology*; and he was Co-Chair of a Euro-American committee which focused on advanced practice in nuclear medicine. Professor Hogg has held several senior academic leadership 'visiting' appointments at various institutions, including Groningen (the

Netherlands), Stockholm (Sweden), Cork (Ireland) and Hong Kong, and he was a Consultant Advisor to the American Society of Radiologic Technologists in the early 2000s. He was also an Honorary Consultant in nuclear medicine in the UK's NHS in the early 2000s. Professor Hogg retired in 2020 and was granted the lifelong title *Professor Emeritus* by the University of Salford's Senate Committee.

Philip Webster qualified in diagnostic radiography and specialised in trauma imaging and information technology, including technical evaluation of Daylight imaging systems, radiology information systems and electronic clinical record structures, and technical assessment of digital imaging and computed tomography scanning systems. He had roles in senior management in acute hospitals and was the UK Department of Health Imaging Technical Lead for 8 years. This role involved supporting a number of service innovations, including oversight of the fast-track magnetic resonance imaging (MRI) programme and leading the initial phase of the programme for the implementation of the NHS proton beam therapy services. As Radiography Advisor to the British Executive Service Overseas (now defunct), a non-governmental organisation, he undertook a number of assignments to support the expansion of radiography practice and imaging services in Poland, North Macedonia and Kenya. He is an Honorary Member of the Royal College of Radiologists and is currently an Advisor on Clinical Research and Molecular Imaging to Alliance Medical Limited.

Louise Kemp is a Diagnostic Radiographer, and an experienced Project and Programme Manager with a varied career in clinical, non-clinical and leadership roles, in both the NHS and the commercial sector. She has extensive experience working in radiology information system (RIS)/ picture archiving and communication system (PACS) management and projects, including working on regional system procurements and implementations. Kemp has also led service improvement projects, developed clinical governance agendas, supported successful Quality Standard for Imaging accreditations and has worked as a radiology service manager. More recently, she has been involved in regional collaborative workforce development projects working with universities and NHS trusts to expand the workforce and increase professional development opportunities for radiographers.

Lesley Wright qualified as a Diagnostic Radiographer, gaining expertise in CT, MRI and nuclear medicine before becoming a Radiology Manager in the north west. Formerly the Director of Diagnostics, NHS Improvement, Wright established the National Radiology Service Improvement team in 2002, and then established the national endoscopy, pathology and cytology improvement programmes, developing and testing improvement techniques, publishing 'how-to' guides and case studies based on evidence-based learning and presenting at national and international improvement forums in the UK, Ireland, the USA and Scandinavia. A qualified Healthcare Systems Engineer (HCSE2) and Lean Six Sigma Black Belt, her focus is to coach clinical teams to embed in-house improvement capability and demonstrate the value that effective and efficient diagnostic services can have across the whole healthcare system.

Contributor

Dr Jo Cresswell is a Research and Knowledge Exchange Consultant and Leadership Coach, entrepreneur and former University Director of Research. With a career spanning nearly 30 years, she has conducted, managed and led research in Russell Group Universities, the National Institute for Health and Care Research and the University of Salford. Dr Cresswell works closely with academic and professional colleagues to create strong research environments and cultures, underpinned by effective, fit-for-purpose research infrastructures, processes and procedures. Over her career, she has delivered a step change in research income and performance, working across disciplines, institutions and sectors. She also specialises in strategy and change development and implementation, working with key internal and external stakeholders to create engagement, buy-in and success.

Series Editor

A. Stewart Whitley served for several years as Directorate Manager for Radiology and Physiotherapy Services at Blackpool Teaching Hospitals NHS Foundation Trust. Following his retirement, he established UK Radiology Advisory Services. Until December 2022, he was the International Society of Radiographers and Radiological Technologists (ISRRT) Director of Professional Practice; prior to that he was the

ISRRT's Treasurer for two terms, serving on several World Health Organization (WHO) and International Atomic Energy Agency (IAEA) committees. He was the radiographers' voice for the Society and College of Radiographers (ScoR) on the working group that formulated the UK Imaging Services Accreditation Scheme (ISAS) – now known as Quality Standards for Imaging. He represented the SCoR on the Pritchard Report committee, which established breast screening in the UK. Whitley is Editor and Series Editor of the Clark's family of radiography textbooks, including *Clark's Positioning in Radiography*, *Clark's Procedures in Diagnostic Imaging* and several 'Clark's Pocket Handbook Guides', covering various topics. He is a Fellow of the College of Radiographers; he was awarded the Society of Radiographers Silver Medal in 2010 and the Gold Medal in May 2022.

ACKNOWLEDGEMENTS

This book would not have been possible without the assistance of many colleagues. First and foremost, we would like to thank Libby Mills, Diagnostics Transformation Programme Manager and Therapeutic Radiographer, who ensured that we were able to deliver content that was appropriate to both diagnostic and therapeutic radiographers.

Numerous people have given their time to support the writing of numerous chapters, whether that is in contributing specialist knowledge or sense-checking to confirm that the work is current and aimed at the correct level for the proposed audience. We would like to thank:

- Fiona Thow for her detailed knowledge on workforce planning;
- Tina Summersgill and David Anwyl for understanding budgets;
- Rachel Hemingway for her endless passion on staff engagement;
- Nancy West for her immense expertise on procurement and managed equipment services in particular;
- Julie Bower for her vast knowledge of informatics and PACS, including in maintaining a service during critical or business continuity incidents.

ABBREVIATIONS

2WW	2-week wait
AAR	after-action review
ACOP	Approved Code of Practice
A-EQUIP	Advocating for Education and QUality ImProvement
AI	artificial intelligence
AL	annual leave
API	aligned payment and incentive approach
BCI	business continuity incident
BI	business intelligence
BSS	basic safety standards
CCG	Clinical Commissioning Group
CDC	Community Diagnostic Centre
CE	Conformité Européenne
CEO	chief executive officer
CI	critical incident
CIP	cost improvement programme
CIPD	Chartered Institute of Personnel and Development
COCIR	Coordination Committee of the Radiological, Electromedical and Healthcare IT Industry
CPD	continuing professional development
CQC	Care Quality Commission
CQI	continuous quality improvement
CT	computed tomography
DHSC	Department of Health and Social Care
DID	Diagnostic Imaging Dataset
DMAIC	define, measure, analyse, improve and control
DNA	did not attend
DPIA	Data Protection Impact Assessment
DPO	data protection officer
DSA	data-sharing agreement
DSPT	Data Security and Protection Toolkit
DVC	Diagnostic Vitals Chart®
ED	Emergency Department
EOI	expression of interest
EPR	electronic patient record

EPRR	emergency preparedness, resilience and response
ESR	European Society of Radiology
EU	European Union
FBC	full business case
FDS	Faster Diagnosis Standard
FFT	Friends and Family Test
FIFO	first in, first out
FOI	freedom of information
FTSU	freedom to speak up
GDPR	General Data Protection Regulation
GIRFT	getting it right first time
GP	general practitioner
GROW	goals, reality, options, will
HCAI	healthcare-associated infection
HCPC	Health and Care Professions Council
HCSE	healthcare systems engineering
HEE	Health Education England
HFMA	Healthcare Financial Management Association
HR	Human Resources
HRG	Healthcare Resource Group
H&S	health and safety
HSA	Health Security Agency
IAEA	International Atomic Energy Agency
ICB	integrated care board
ICO	Information Commissioner's Office
ICP	integrated care partnership
ICS	integrated care system
ID	identifier or identification
IG	information governance
IP	inpatient
IPC	infection prevention and control
IRMER	Ionising Radiation (Medical Exposure) Regulations 2017
IRR	Ionising Radiations Regulations
IRR (NI)	Ionising Radiations Regulations (Northern Ireland)
ISRRT	International Society of Radiographers and Radiological Technologists
IT	information technology
ITT	invite to tender
JD	job description
KLOE	key line of enquiry
KPI	key performance indicator

Abbreviations

LFPSE	Learn From Patient Safety Events
LPA	laser protection advisor
LPS	laser protection supervisor
MDT	multidisciplinary team
MES	managed equipment service
MHRA	Medicines and Healthcare products Regulatory Agency
MHS	Model Health System
MI	major incident
MP	Member of Parliament
MPE	medical physics expert
MPI	master patient index
MRI	magnetic resonance imaging
NHSBSA	NHS Business Services Authority
NHSE	NHS England
NHSI	NHS Improvement
NHSPS	NHS Payment Scheme
NHSR	NHS Resolution
NHSTD	NHS England Transformation Directorate
NICE	National Institute for Health and Care Excellence
NIHR	National Institute for Health and Care Research
NIPCM	National Infection Prevention and Control Manual
NPSA	National Patient Safety Alerts
NRLS	National Reporting and Learning System
OAR	organ at risk
OBC	outline business case
OCRR	Order Communications and Results Reporting
OH	occupational health
OP	operating procedure
OPD	Outpatient Department
OPM	Office of Personnel Management
PACS	picture archiving and communication system
PALS	Patient Advice and Liaison Service
PAS	patient administration system
PBP	place-based partnership
PDP	personal development plan
PDSA	plan, do, study, act
PhD	Doctor of Philosophy
PIN	prior information notice
PPE	personal protective equipment
PPM	planned preventative maintenance
PS	person specification
PSII	patient safety incident investigation

PSIRF	Patient Safety Incident Response Framework
QA	quality assurance
QC	quality control
QSIR	quality, service improvement and redesign
RBAC	role-based access controls
RIS	radiology information system
RPA	radiation protection advisor
RPS	radiation protection supervisor
RTDS	Radiotherapy Data Set
RVS	record-and-verify system
RWA	radioactive waste advisor
SEIPS	System Engineering Initiative for Patient Safety
SFI	Standing Financial Instruction
SFQP	safety, flow, quality and productivity
SIRO	senior information risk owner
SMART	specific, measurable, achievable, relevant and time-bound
SOC	strategic outline case
SOP	standard operating procedure
SoR	Society of Radiographers
SPC	statistical process control
StEIS	Strategic Executive Information System
TIMWOODS	transport, inventory, motion, waiting, overproduction, overprocessing, defects and skills
TL	time in lieu
TTBACO	time traps, batching and carve-out
UCL	upper control limit
UKCA	UK Conformity Assessed
WHO	World Health Organization
WIP	work in progress
WLI	waiting list initiative
WTE	whole-time equivalent

SECTION 1
INTRODUCTION

1. LEADERSHIP IN HEALTHCARE

Amanda Martin, Jo Cresswell and Peter Hogg

INTRODUCTION

In June 2022, Sir Gordon Messenger produced a report on the NHS, Leadership for a Collaborative and Inclusive Future.[1] The purpose of the report was to examine the state of leadership and management in the NHS and social care sector. While recognising the high quality of leadership within the UK NHS, it makes seven key recommendations:

1. targeted interventions on collaborative leadership and organisational values;
2. positive equality, diversity and inclusion;
3. consistent management standards delivered through accredited training;
4. a simplified, standard appraisal system;
5. a new career and talent management function for the senior leadership teams;
6. more effective recruitment and development of non-executive directors;
7. encouraging top talent into challenged parts of the system.

In addition, the recent Richards report, Diagnostics: Recovery and Renewal (October 2020), has set a new direction for diagnostics and radiology, requiring radical change for the delivery of radiology services.[2] This document, commissioned by NHS England, demonstrated the need for radical investment and reform of diagnostic services in England. The publication makes the case for change, with 24 recommendations and actions focusing on seven key themes (**Figure 1.1**).

                                    DOI: 9781003380078-1

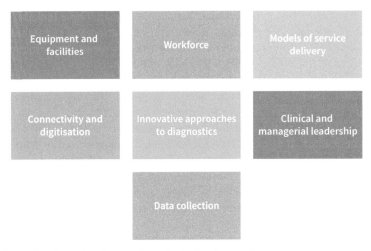

Figure 1.1 Seven key themes from the Richards report.

It has set the direction for radiology via 28 **imaging networks**. Implementation of the recommendations will help drive improved outcomes in cancer, stroke, heart disease, respiratory disease and other conditions. We highly recommend reading this document as a foundation to understand the new direction and radical change for radiology services that will be delivered by the new imaging networks. This new direction requires excellent local management and leadership for it to be successful, with the recommendations of the Messenger report being key to this.

Management is concerned with how goals are achieved through the effective organisation of people, physical resources and activities.[3] To help achieve this, managers are appointed into jobs at varying levels within organisations. Leadership can be seen in two ways. First is leaders as holders of senior jobs within organisations. Employees holding such positions are often responsible for setting organisational strategy and, through the senior leadership team and others, ensuring such strategy is implemented. They might also be senior clinical employees, for example consultant radiographers, a concept first introduced in 1999 by the Department of Health[4] where clinicians combine clinical expertise with management and leadership roles. Second, leadership can be ·

3

seen as a set of behavioural traits that people display. These include, for example, emotion, empathy, authenticity, innovation and adaptability, and the ability to inspire others. Such behaviours mean that things can get done effectively and efficiently with and through others.

Anybody can display leadership behaviours and thus be classified as a leader. Therefore, you do not need to be part of the senior leadership team to be a leader. Junior radiographers through to the chief executive can all display leadership behaviours and, in doing so, they will all be leaders. It is expected that radiology managers, senior leaders, consultant and advanced practice radiographers and superintendent/lead radiographers will exhibit leadership behaviours; otherwise they will be less effective in their jobs. However, while a manager must also be a leader, it is not necessarily so that a person in a formal leadership role must be a manager.

A manager maintains status quo and stability while determining the aims of the service, and uses management tools, such as project/business planning, to facilitate achievement of these aims. A leader sets the direction and remit of the plans and facilitates change by influencing, inspiring and motivating individuals to works towards achieving the aims.

It might be possible to manage without having well-developed leadership skills, but this may bring challenges in moving the organisation forward. It is possible to lead without management skills, but any changes may not be sustained if nobody is managing that change. Management and leadership are inherently different; both are complementary aspects of some roles. While managing people can be effective in stable times, in times of instability, such as those caused by the rapid changes within the NHS, management alone is not enough, and people need to be led.

Often, radiographers find themselves in a new job or taking on a new role that requires them to have well-defined, and perhaps quite advanced, leadership behaviours; however, they might have had very little preparation for this and, as a result, could struggle. For example, a newly promoted (senior) radiographer may have a role in their job that makes them responsible for a small team delivering a specific element of the service within radiology. Or it might be that no promotion is involved, but the radiographer takes on a new role, such as roster planning or conducting sickness absence reviews. In both cases, they would need to have suitably developed leadership behaviours to help them fulfil the responsibility.

At this point, it is worth mentioning that a radiographer can start to develop leadership behaviours quite soon in their career, whether or not they want to progress down a route that demands them as part of a job person specification or job role. The best leaders are ones who model and seek to instil good leadership behaviours in all team members, regardless of banding or career stage. Jobs that require good leadership behaviours include management appointments, senior clinical posts (e.g. consultant radiographer/advanced practitioner) and academic appointments (e.g. teacher and/or researcher).

OVERVIEW OF LEADERSHIP STYLES, MODELS AND THEORIES

There are as many definitions of leadership as there are models and theories. Adair (2002) proposes that leadership is about taking people on a journey towards a common vision.[5] The idea of taking people on a journey suggests that effective leadership is not a lonely experience, but an adventure consisting of new encounters to be shared with others. A substantial body of literature has been published about leadership behaviours, styles, models and theories. Simply search publishing company websites or e-commerce company search engines, such as Amazon, and you will find a vast range of leadership books. Such texts can be focused on a particular leadership theory, they could have a broader multi-theory approach or they might be written to specific subsections of society (e.g. female leaders). After reading this chapter, if you remain interested in developing your leadership abilities, we recommend strongly that you select suitable additional reading materials to enhance your understanding of leadership; selection of such materials would be best done with the support of a mentor as they can guide you to select the most appropriate materials suited to you and your context.

Leadership theories have been developed through observational studies over many decades and aim to explain why some people make good leaders, with some focusing on essential characteristics while others explore behaviours. There are many leadership theories, and these include the following:

- The Great Man theory was developed in the 19th century (hence the emphasis on gender). This suggests that leaders are born with the required skills and those skills cannot be learnt; it is similar to trait theory, which suggests that leadership is a natural talent that is either present or absent within an individual. Neither differentiate between good and bad leaders, nor do they address interactions between leader and employee.
- Behavioural theory is the opposite of Great Man theory in that it proposes that leaders can be made: people can learn leadership skills and demonstrate good leadership through their learned actions rather than their intrinsic skills.
- Transactional theory demonstrates a hierarchical approach with a directive manner embedded within a robust structure and using reward and punishment to achieve goals. At its extreme, this manifests as an authoritarian leader who directs the team, making unilateral decisions without any collaboration.
- Contingency theory indicates that a leader may be effective in one situation, but not in a different situation. Awareness of where their skills lie and in what situations they may feel challenged will enable leaders to focus on their own development. Similarly, situational theory emphasises the ability to lead dependent on the situation, but, in this instance, the leader has the ability to adapt their style to the given situation or the abilities of those around them.
- Participative theory focuses on the democratic leader who allows their team members to contribute to decision-making, but makes the final decision, albeit with consideration of others' input.
- Transformational theory is perhaps the most relevant within modern healthcare. This has a substantial focus on interactions between individuals; the leader demonstrates visionary skills and, through influencing and encouragement, is able to inspire others to achieve a common goal. They are attentive to others and motivate them to achieve. They encourage problem-solving and development by inspiring others to do the right thing for the team rather than for themselves as an individual. Transformational leaders encourage team members to challenge their own beliefs.

More recently, new models of leadership are being built on the foundations of these theories, allowing more relevance to the opportunities, challenges, and societal and cultural influences of the 21st century. These include servant, innovative, pace-setting, charismatic and laissez-faire models of leadership.

In a large organisation, a collective leadership culture is most effective as this recognises differing expertise and acknowledges that the leader may change dependent on the situation. However, each leader in that organisation will have their own leadership style.

There are four general leadership styles: **directive**, **coaching**, **participative** and **delegation**; each is used in different models of leadership and all of them can be beneficial in specific circumstances. Indeed, there needs to be flexibility within all leaders so that the correct style is used based on the task and team. Recognising which style and which behavioural traits to use in differing situations will enable you to have a wider view of the challenges, communicate more effectively and develop people and teams to achieve desired outcomes and shared goals.

TRAITS AND BEHAVIOURS OF EFFECTIVE LEADERS

In this section of the chapter, we identify and explain some leadership behavioural traits that have been published in the literature and that we believe are especially valuable for radiographers who wish to develop their leadership abilities. In some respects, good leadership behaviours can be viewed as simply being nice to others. When people are nice to others, they tend to be liked by others and this can result in things getting done by them and by those around them. The first seven leadership traits can be achieved by anybody, irrespective of grade or profession.

1. *Have a positive impact on others.* This can be achieved in many ways, so consider being creative when addressing this point. Examples of helpful behaviours include thanking people when they have done something, praising them for doing something well or even praising them for having a go at doing something difficult. Simple things, such as offering to make tea or coffee

for others, can make others feel good about you and themselves. If you have a few spare minutes and somebody working near you appears to be struggling or is overly rushed or stressed, then consider offering some help.

2. *Value others.* This is related to point 1; doing this makes people feel good about themselves and the contribution they make. Consider taking a broad view on this, instead of focusing purely on the technicalities of their work, and take a moment to consider how *they* would feel most valued. Examples include telling others that the work they are doing is great and that you appreciate them as a professional, telling others (especially their senior leaders) that they are a considerate person and that you like working with them and telling them that activities that they do in their social life (e.g. charitable activities) are important and valuable and you appreciate what they do for people in that context.

3. *Promote teamwork.* Teams are more effective than individuals, in terms of the amount and quality of work that can be achieved. When working in teams there are a lot of social and psychological factors to consider, to ensure the team is effective. These factors include reflecting critically on yourself, with regard to your contribution to the team's objectives and goals, how you are perceived by others and how you perceive others in the context of team working. Personal reflection could result in you making changes to your behaviour, with a view to improving your contribution to team working. There is a huge body of literature on teams, and we encourage you to read widely on this topic and to reflect and implement changes to your own style if needed.

4. *Invite feedback from others about you and your style, listen carefully to what is said and make changes as needed.* Adopting a critical and reflective approach can improve your leadership skills and it should heighten your value in a team. We should offer a word of caution about soliciting feedback from others – the process can be painful, as you might hear things you do not want to hear. Rather than being reactive to negative feedback, take the time to reflect and to understand the reasons underpinning the feedback. The actions that follow negative feedback are often the ones that allow greater growth. Go back and

ask for further feedback once your actions are complete. This is a cycle of learning and developing into a competent leader.

5. *Build relationships with others.* We have already mentioned that teams are more effective than individuals and that people work well with others when they know and like them. Therefore, consider getting to know people who you work with and even start to get to know others in your work environment who you might end up working with. For the former, assuming others are comfortable doing this, it could simply involve engaging colleagues in conversations about their personal lives (e.g. hobbies, family). For the latter, it could involve sitting with people you do not know in shared social workspaces and involving them in conversations about work and non-work topics. In both instances it might be helpful if there is some work-related discussion when building professional relationships around shared/common interests. It may also be beneficial to start networking with others who may impact on your future career development, for example attendance at multidisciplinary team meetings within your own organisation or attendance at a local study day where other attendees have succeeded in their own development.

6. *Use effective communication styles.* Communication is a two-way process – listening to others and conveying information to them. Once again, a considerable body of literature has been published on how you can be effective at both. There is an art to being an effective listener, and being an effective listener heightens your chance of understanding what others are saying, as well as demonstrating to others that you are interested in what they are saying. By employing active listening skills – such as attentive body language and asking clarifying questions – the person communicating with you can recognise instantly that you are interested and often they will respond to these positive cues. This gives them confidence and often improves their communication performance. It is worthwhile reading about active listening, including verbal and non-verbal techniques that can be used to enhance your listening skills as perceived by the person communicating with you. Obviously, a range of media can be used in communication, going beyond face-to-face communication. Your ability to write coherently, succinctly and in a non-offensive

9

fashion will be critical and needs to be employed in professional emails and in report writing; therefore, it is important to pause and reflect on how your written communication might be received by your audience. Again, development opportunities do exist for improving your written English as well as etiquette in written and verbal communication in different contexts and forums.

7. ***Do what you say you will do.*** This point relates to your integrity and reliability. If you agree to do something, then do it and do it within the agreed time frame. Others around you will depend upon you to play your part in a timely fashion. Not following through with something you agreed to do places an unnecessary burden of responsibility and pressure on the person or people that you agreed to support/do something for. Of course, there will be circumstances when you may not be able to meet your commitments, but these circumstances should be limited to 'the unexpected', such as illness.

While the above can be developed and demonstrated by anybody, the next behaviours are normally associated with those holding more senior positions.

8. ***Develop capability in others.*** Good leaders develop those around them; this might involve identifying or even creating opportunities for others to gain experience and skills. Capability can be developed through supporting others to attend formal programmes of study, from 1-day events to those lasting a few years (such as a master's degree). Capability can also be developed by allocating tasks to others, perhaps by devolving activities or parts of activities from your own portfolio of professional responsibilities, or by inviting ideas from others and, where appropriate, giving them the space to explore these ideas further. Developing others concerns much more than giving somebody a job to do or sending them on a study programme. It should also involve formal and informal interactions with them, in a coaching or mentorship capacity, to help them with the learning process and to give them constructive feedback on their development and performance. Importantly, through coaching or mentorship, developing others should continually be linked to the job they are currently doing;

it is also valuable to link their development to how it will impact any future career ambitions they might have.

9. *Give staff freedom to act, but support them and provide them with feedback for improvement.* If you allocate a responsibility or task to a member of your team, avoid micromanagement and allow them a chance to do the work as independently as possible and to report back to you when it has been done. As needed, you should offer support to them, but consider allowing them the freedom to come back to you for help and guidance when they feel they need to. You must take a leap of faith in the member of staff when taking this approach, as you are placing a belief in them that they can do what is required, and if they cannot, that they will come back to you as needed. If you take this approach, you must be prepared for them to make mistakes. This being the case, you should have risk-assessed the task they are to do and have put in place adequate mitigation as needed. Importantly, mistakes should be viewed as learning opportunities and you should give helpful, constructive and supportive feedback when mistakes occur. In the event of them completing a task extremely well, you should still give feedback and explain why the task was done well. It can help to follow the golden rule of giving credit for successes and taking ultimate responsibility when things do not go according to plan – this creates trust and psychological safety, which are critical for effective leadership.

10. *Involve colleagues.* Too often people believe that it is easier or better to do the task by themselves. Justifications for this approach can include a perception that it will take longer to train others to do the task or citing times when others have let them down previously and/or have produced work that did not meet their personal standards. The challenge is that, as a leader, this will result in you being less effective on the tasks that only you can do. When you do not delegate, you may fail to acknowledge the benefits to the organisation of involving others, harnessing new ideas and perspectives and, importantly, the fact that effective teams can produce better outcomes and higher volumes of outputs than individuals working in isolation. Involving others allows the continual development of team members, which has many benefits, including continuity should a key member of staff

leave the organisation. Involving others can also inspire others to develop and to go on and achieve improved outcomes as time progresses. Involving others is also a way of valuing people, which was mentioned earlier.

11. ***Inspire a shared purpose within your team.*** Most radiographers will work within teams, even if that team is located remotely. Whether the radiographer works for the NHS or private health-care, the organisation will have strategic ambitions. Such ambitions impact all staff within the organisation and teams are formed to play their part in helping to achieve the required outcomes. Team members should be fully aware of organisational strategic ambitions and how their team's work relates to helping achieve organisational ambitions. Each team should have a clear purpose and all team members should be aware of that purpose and how their individual input contributes to the team's purpose and outcomes. Teams should work in an interdependent fashion, with each member relying on other members to play their parts in order to make an effective whole that has a common purpose.

12. ***Create and lead effective teams.*** People in senior positions are likely to have team-related responsibilities; these could include creating and leading effective teams. When creating a team, it is important that team members are selected on the skills they possess, such that when individual skills are taken as a collective, they should match what is needed to achieve the team outcomes. However, there will be many occasions when you must include people in your team who do not possess the right skills at the outset. In this case, it is important to select people who have shown that they can learn and grow within a team. Such people can be an asset, as they bring new perspectives; however, you will need to help develop their abilities to the required levels – as mentioned earlier in this chapter. Leading a team is an active process and does not simply involve telling the team what needs to be done. It will also involve managing interpersonal relation-ships and individual personalities, to ensure harmony occurs within the team so that working conditions are conducive to the production of outcomes that meet required quality standards. To achieve this, you must have good communication skills and, in

addition, you may find yourself having to be a good negotiator or even arbitrator.

13. ***Strategic influencing.*** This is a critical leadership skill that has two main elements. First, you may want or need to influence those higher up the management chain and in more senior positions than you. For example, you may want to put a proposal to senior leaders that will enable you, your team or the organisation to achieve a better outcome. Achieving this is made easier when you have a good working relationship with those senior leaders, and they respect your opinions and abilities. In this circumstance an informal conversation or a polite request might suffice. However, if you suspect that senior leaders may not be supportive or may not understand the relevance or benefits of your proposal to the organisation, then a more formal elaborate approach might be required, and the use of strategic influencing methods would be beneficial. Second, you may wish to influence people who do not report to you, or do not have any professional accountability towards you. These people may be within your own organisation, external stakeholders, service users or other people outside your organisation. For example, you or your teams may work on multi-professional teams that include people from other organisations. In this case, using levers of influence such as reciprocity, commitment, consistency and liking is a powerful strategy. For example, when you need support from others, ensure that you have a friendly relationship. Offer to support them in return, and ensure you follow through. In either case, building excellent, trusted, reciprocal relationships with people within your organisation is critical to enabling you to influence strategically.

14. ***Show people what success looks like.*** This is important: teams and individuals will benefit from seeing what a suitable/good outcome is, as this gives them a level and goal to aim for. It can also help motivate them to achieve the success that needs to be achieved. 'Show' might not be a physical representation; it could be communicated through feedback, highlighting the success of others or setting personal or team objectives. It is vital to acknowledge and give credit for success both to guide future actions and to show employees that their contribution is valued.

15. ***Influencing for results.*** Influencing others is essential in effecting change. This is not about forcing your agenda and disregarding the views of others, but is about you being able to eloquently articulate an alternative perspective that improves understanding and encourages others to think differently. Influential leaders are inspirational and motivate others to achieve a common goal; this may be staff who are more junior or senior to you within the organisation. To be effective, you need to build relationships based on trust and credibility, and you need to support and encourage others to make informed decisions collaboratively, rather than dominate the decision-making process. Organisational knowledge will help in directing your influencing skills by identifying those people who may be key to supporting change.

16. ***Evaluating information.*** Critical evaluation skills are vital for leaders at all levels, especially so for those at more senior levels. You should be able and prepared to take an objective, independent view on any information presented. This enables you to be more effective at decision-making, strategy development, resolution of issues and long-term planning. When given any information, it is important for you to check where the information has come from and when it was produced. Is it from a reliable source, and up to date? If the information is supporting an argument, do the numbers or statements back this up? If a proposal is being put forward, with performance expectations, does the information presented support the likelihood of these claims? When it comes to inter-staff or performance matters, you should make efforts to ensure you are aware and can take account of all relevant information to resolve issues and properly address performance.

17. ***Connecting our service.*** There are many different teams working in health and social care; when these teams work independently of each other, this can result in different visions and goals and a lack of cohesiveness within the patient journey. There is an interdependent relationship between most teams, and you need to understand where your team fits into the system to ensure continuity of service for the patient. Effective relationships across teams, and knowledge of the stakeholders associated with each team – patients, referrers, suppliers, for example – is essential so

that decisions can be made that meet the needs of stakeholders, but do not negatively impact other interdependent teams.

18. ***Creating clarity of expectations.*** Clear, unambiguous communication is required so that there is no misunderstanding of the message that is being conveyed. Ambiguity and misunderstandings result in failure to meet goals, either individual performance goals or organisational targets. When defining expectations, whether that is in a job description or an appraisal, for example, these should be delivered in an open and transparent way that is jargon free and, therefore, easily understood by all.

19. ***Holding to account.*** Despite being supportive of colleagues and team members, there will be times when people do not produce work of a suitable standard and/or within an agreed timescale. In these situations, a clear and objective conversation will need to be held between you and your colleague in which you explore why this situation has occurred. Depending on what is said, clear performance expectations may be needed, along with the steps you and they will need to take to ensure the issue will not happen again. It is important to note that there may be many reasons why a colleague or team member may not be performing to the standard required, and compassion may be needed. For example, the individual may be experiencing a significant personal issue – such as illness of a close friend or family member – which is causing issues with their performance. A sign of this can be if performance suddenly declines. If this is the case, then it is incumbent upon you, as team leader, to gain the individual's trust and confidence such that they will feel able to talk with you about the issue and what support they need, and that they will come to you immediately for support if they encounter a similar problem in the future. Alternatively, it might be that they fail to perform adequately due to lack of skills, for which you might support further development for them. It might be that they lack motivation and a conversation will be needed to understand why, and what support or additional responsibility might help to re-energise them. Clear expectations on performance and actions the individual must take (and when), plus the consequences of not meeting these standards, are vital in any discussions around

performance. Ultimately, it could be that, despite your efforts and support as a team leader, the individual is not able to perform at the required level, in which case you would need to involve your organisation's Human Resources department for advice and support on what to do, including putting the individual through a formal performance management process.

DEVELOPING LEADERSHIP ABILITIES

Leadership development, resulting in good leaders, needs to be embedded into organisations to enable growth in individuals, teams and organisations. Most people are not born with highly developed leadership traits, so development is usually needed to engender effective leadership behaviours. Not surprisingly, following development, some people will be better at displaying effective leadership behaviours than others; such differences could be due to the quality of learning provided, inherent abilities and/or the leader's internal self-concept (how they view themselves based on the beliefs they hold about themselves and others).

Various options exist to help with developing or improving your leadership ability and confidence; these range from reflective self-directed to attending a formal programme of study that includes practical and theoretical assessments. One size will not fit all, and you will need to decide which suits your needs best. The simplest option is reflective self-directed, which requires you to engage in reading, put ideas into practice and then to reflect on your experiences while considering the views of others on your abilities. While self-directed is the cheapest option, its limitations include there being no validated certification of your abilities – which might limit career progression at job interviews.

Many leadership programmes exist, offered by private educational and management companies, colleges, universities and the NHS itself. In addition, professional organisations may offer schemes to support new leaders, such as the leadership mentoring scheme offered by the Society of Radiographers.[6] Such programmes might be short (e.g. 6 months) through to a complete master's degree of a few years' duration. The NHS offers a range of leadership development opportunities; these can be seen on the NHS Leadership Academy website.[7] In addition, your own organisation most likely offers leadership training that has numerous stages for progression based on an individual's own development. These may be aimed at different levels of leadership, for example those entering their first-line management role, or at different groups of staff, such as ethnically diverse employees. If you have not experienced any leadership training, your organisation may be a good first place to start. 'E-learning for healthcare' modules[8] have also been developed to support those on their leadership journeys. Good leadership programmes will include a broad range of topics, including, but not limited to:

- problem-solving;
- working with others;
- leading change;
- coaching skills;
- performance management;
- facilitating learning in the workplace.

The NHS Leadership Academy website also contains the healthcare leadership model, which includes the nine leadership dimensions. The model is a self-help online document that helps you improve your leadership abilities in the context of healthcare/the NHS. It helps you to reflect on your own behaviours to help you decide if your leadership skills are adequate for the post you occupy. Overall, it is generally repackaged material from various other published theories under headings suitable for jobs in care settings. Ideally, you should use it alongside other leadership literature sources. It also provides useful practical tips, and it includes practically related questions that can help shape your leadership behaviours. Ideally, you should use it under the guidance of a mentor. A 360-degree appraisal for leadership would be beneficial to do at various points of your development. This will enable you to assess your leadership abilities/behaviours and identify your strengths and areas for development. Over time, you should see improvement, and this should be reflected in your day-to-day practices, with improved team motivation, engagement and performance. Leadership theories often change and so it is important not to follow or rely on any single model as it will evolve, or even be replaced, as time progresses; you should keep abreast of such changes.

CHAPTER SUMMARY

- Management is concerned with how goals are achieved through the effective organisation of people, physical resources and activities.
- Leaders set organisational strategy and, through managers, ensure it is implemented.
- The best leaders model and instil good leadership behaviours in all team members.
- Many leadership theories have been developed over the years. Transformational leadership is the most relevant to the healthcare setting.
- Understanding leadership behaviours and traits is essential for those wishing to develop their leadership skills.
- The four leadership styles are directive, coaching, participative and delegation; recognising which style to use in a given situation will enable you to have a wider view of the challenges, communicate more effectively and develop people and teams to achieve desired outcomes and shared goals.
- Within a large organisation, a collective leadership culture is most effective as this recognises differing expertise and acknowledges that the leader may change dependent on the situation.

FURTHER READING

- Cialdini, R. *Influence: The Psychology of Persuasion*. New York: HarperCollins; 2007.
- Kouses, J.M. and Posner B.Z. *The Leadership Challenge: How to Make Extraordinary Things Happen in Organizations*. Hoboken: Wiley; 2023.
- NHS England and Health Education England. Leadership Development. 2018. Available at www.england.nhs.uk/wp-content/uploads/2018/03/leadership-development.pdf.

- Salt, T. *Effective Leadership in Health and Social Care: Towards Outstanding Teams and Services.* Shoreham-by-Sea: Pavilion Publishing and Media Ltd; 2022.

REFERENCES

1. Messenger, G. and Pollard, L. Leadership for a Collaborative and Inclusive Future. 2022. Available at www.gov.uk/government/publications/health-and-social-care-review-leadership-for-a-collaborative-and-inclusive-future.
2. Richards, M. Diagnostics: Recovery and Renewal. 2020. Available at www.england.nhs.uk/publication/diagnostics-recovery-and-renewal-report-of-the-independent-review-of-diagnostic-services-for-nhs-england/.
3. Liphadzi, M., Aigbavboa, C.O. and Thwala, W.D. A theoretical perspective on the difference between leadership and management. *Procedia Engineering* 2017;**196**:478–482. From the Creative Construction Conference 2017 (CCC 2017), 19–22 June 2017, Primošten, Croatia.
4. Department of Health. *Making a Difference.* London: Stationery Office; 1999.
5. Adair, J. *Effective Strategic Leadership.* London: Macmillan; 2002.
6. Society of Radiographers. Career Development. Available at www.sor.org/learning-advice/career-development.
7. NHS Leadership Academy. Available at www.leadershipacademy.nhs.uk.
8. NHS England. Elearning for Healthcare. Available at https://portal.e-lfh.org.uk/Login.

2. HEALTH AND SOCIAL CARE STRUCTURES

Amanda Martin and Lesley Wright

INTRODUCTION

The delivery of health and social care services requires multiple, and often complex, organisations to work together. This is funded through taxation and is mainly free at the point of care to all UK nationals; other countries may supplement this with the requirement for private health insurance, and some countries rely solely on private health insurance as the only means of accessing healthcare. It is not possible to review global healthcare structures in detail and this chapter will focus on the NHS in the UK. The NHS encompasses many organisations responsible for different elements of healthcare service; these will be introduced in this chapter. While the focus will be on the English NHS, the organisations mentioned are also embedded in the other three UK nations and, although their names may be different, their aims are the same (**Figure 2.1**). Information provided here is accurate at the time of writing. Due to the fast-changing nature of health and social care, web addresses have been included so that you can undertake further reading and check for current information.

DOI: 9781003380078-2

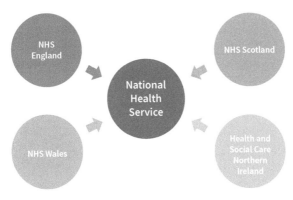

Figure 2.1 The nations making up the NHS.

FUNDING MODEL FOR THE NHS

The budget for the NHS is determined by the UK government on an annual basis and is taken from money raised through:

- taxation;
- National Insurance payments;
- prescription charges;
- general ophthalmic services;
- charges for dental treatment.

Funding is distributed to the health and care providers in different ways, dependent on the nation, but primarily through national bodies in each nation in the UK (**Figure 2.2**). These government bodies are responsible for:

- leading the delivery of national healthcare services in their nation;
- setting strategy;
- commissioning services such as general practitioners (GPs), dentists and pharmacists.[1]

Their focus is on health promotion and protection, improving social care provision and delivering better healthcare outcomes. Through horizon scanning, they can anticipate future health and social care needs and put plans in place to address them.

21

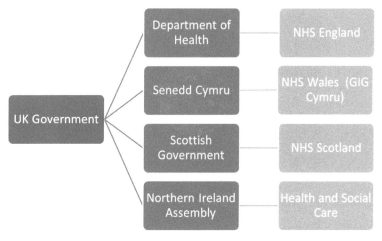

Figure 2.2 Flow of funding in the UK nations.

NHS ENGLAND

NHS England (NHSE) is the senior decision-making structure for the NHS in England. In recent years, NHSE has seen several mergers, with NHS Improvement (NHSI) merging in 2022 and NHS Digital and Health Education England merging in 2023. As a result, NHSE is now responsible for setting strategic direction and overseeing its delivery for health and social care in England, training and education of the workforce, national information technology (IT) systems and data and driving clinical improvements. Around 85% of the government funding passes from NHSE to **integrated care boards** (ICBs) for direct patient care, with the remainder being used for training and development, regulation and public health activities. The ICB makes decisions on spending the money based on local need. This could be within primary, secondary or tertiary care and may include improvements to local health and social care facilities, operations and treatments that they will fund and services that they will commission. This money is then passed on to the providers who deliver the required services. This function was previously carried out by Clinical Commissioning Groups (CCGs). A similar system operates in Wales, Scotland and Northern

Ireland, where there are geographical health boards that plan, commission and deliver NHS services in their respective localities.

The ICB is part of an **integrated care system** (ICS), a partnership of organisations with the following purposes:

- to work together to plan and deliver joined-up health and care services;
- to improve outcomes in population health and healthcare and to improve the lives of people who live and work in their area;
- to tackle inequalities in outcomes, experience and access;
- to enhance productivity and value for money;
- to help the NHS to support broader social and economic development.

Established in 2022 following publication of the Health and Care Act (2022),[2,3] there are 42 ICSs in England, with each comprising an ICB and an **integrated care partnership** (ICP), a statutory committee jointly formed between the NHS ICB and all upper-tier local authorities within the ICS area that are responsible for social care and public health functions, as well as other vital services for local people and businesses. The ICP sets the strategic direction for meeting the health and care needs of the local population. The detailed design and delivery of these services is led by place-based partnerships (PBPs), which involve many representatives from the NHS, local councils, residents and community and voluntary organisations.

SUPPORTING ORGANISATIONS

The English NHS is made up of many organisations that support service delivery. Many of these are classed as executive organisations, meaning that they are part of the Department of Health and Social Care structure, but, managerially and financially, they work independently. While there are too many to mention in this book, below is a summary of the role of the more significant ones.

Care Quality Commission

Every organisation providing health and/or social care services must be registered with the Care Quality Commission (CQC). It is an independent regulator responsible for ensuring that high-quality health and social care is provided that is effective, safe and compassionate. There are five standards against which an organisation or service is assessed. Is it:

1. safe?
2. effective?
3. caring?
4. responsive?
5. well-led?

Each of the above standards has several quality statements within it and these are used to measure the outcomes of a service during an inspection. Inspections take place either on-site or through other means, such as data collection, focus groups or submitted evidence. These can be planned as part of a scheduled inspection programme or can be in response to a concern that may have been raised. The whole organisation may not be inspected in the latter case – a focused inspection is more likely to take place.

Once an inspection has taken place, a rating is given: **inadequate**, **requires improvement**, **good** or **outstanding**. These ratings are given for each standard and then an overall rating is given. If one of the standards receives an inadequate rating, then an action plan is required, and a re-inspection of that standard will take place within 6 months. If no improvement has been made in that standard, or if the overall rating is inadequate, then the organisation will be put into special measures to protect those who use their services. This involves the development of a detailed plan for improvement in conjunction with NHSE and identifying sources for support and guidance prior to a re-inspection in 6 months. The CQC can also use enforcement powers such as imposing conditions of registration, issuing warning notices or removing registration completely.

More information can be accessed at *www.cqc.org.uk*.

Health Security Agency

In April 2021, Public Health England was replaced by the UK Health Security Agency (HSA); it is responsible for protecting the public from the impact of harmful diseases or substances in England.

More information can be accessed at *www.gov.uk/government/ organisations/uk-health-security-agency.*

Imaging Networks

In 2019, NHSE published 'Transforming Imaging Services in England: A National Strategy for Imaging Networks'.[4] This strategy led to 22 collaborative diagnostic imaging networks being established across England. The networks are based on a geographical footprint and on patient flows for a range of conditions including cancer, stroke, major trauma, acute cardiology and maternity services. It was developed to address the challenges that are being faced across radiology with increased demand and shortages in the workforce, as well as old equipment impacting on the ability to deliver efficient services. To support them, a series of guidance documents have been published that focus on implementation, workforce, capital equipment planning and commercial structure and operational governance. The benefits of the networks are as follows:

- a cohesive approach to quality improvement across imaging networks;
- improved sustainability and service resilience;
- staffing consistency and flexibility, supporting enhanced personal development;
- staff retention through flexible working and flexible retirement opportunities;
- sharing and levelling of resources for both staff and equipment;
- economies of scale in procurement for both capital equipment and outsourcing services;
- reducing unwarranted financial variation of both pay and non-pay costs;
- ensuring equal access for all patients, irrespective of geography;
- locally acquired images, with distributed reporting networks, which allows access to sub-specialty opinion, irrespective of location;
- shared capacity and management of imaging reporting backlogs to optimise reporting turnaround times;
- management of outsourcing and insourcing in a planned and financially sustainable way;
- maintaining high-quality learning and training environments.

25

Medicines and Healthcare Products Regulatory Agency

The Medicines and Healthcare products Regulatory Agency (MHRA) is responsible for the standards associated with medicines, medical devices (including radiology and radiotherapy equipment) and blood components for transfusion. It makes sure that, for example, radiology equipment meets the quality and safety standards and is suitable and safe for use in a clinical environment. It is responsible for issuing licences for new drugs or devices.

More information can be accessed at *www.gov.uk/government/organisations/medicines-and-healthcare-products-regulatory-agency*.

National Institute for Health and Care Excellence

The National Institute for Health and Care Excellence (NICE) is responsible for much of the evidence-based practice that takes place across health and social care, with the aim being to provide national guidance and advice to improve outcomes. There are numerous NICE guidelines that outline best practice and help service providers to deliver the highest standard of care to patients. While not legally binding, there is an expectation that they will be followed, and organisations are often audited on practice against NICE guidelines.

More information can be accessed at *www.nice.org.uk*.

National Institute for Health and Care Research

The National Institute for Health and Care Research (NIHR) funds and delivers research that is beneficial to health and social care. It also provides support and education to health and care in the following ways:

- specialist career development support;
- providing new knowledge and skills with learning tools to help health and care professionals in research improve care for patients and the public;
- providing the latest evidence in research;

- encouraging patients and service users to get involved in research studies.

More information can be accessed at *www.nihr.ac.uk*.

NHS Business Services Authority

The NHS Business Services Authority (NHSBSA) delivers a wide range of services to NHS organisations and contractors, patients and the public. Examples of these services are NHS pensions, prescription prepayment certificates and funding for health and social care training.

More information can be accessed at *www.nhsbsa.nhs.uk*.

NHS England Transformation Directorate

In 2019, NHSX was launched to support local organisations in delivering the digital agenda, before integrating into the NHS England Transformation Directorate (NHSTD) in 2022. The prime focus is on driving digital transformation within health and social care. Within NHSTD is the NHS Artificial Intelligence Laboratory, which involves experts from academia and technology researching the use of artificial intelligence (AI) in health and care settings.

More information can be accessed at *https://transform.england.nhs.uk/*.

NHS Resolution

Previously called NHS Litigation Authority, NHS Resolution (NHSR) deals with compensation claims made against an NHS organisation and advises on concerns raised about the performance of an individual practitioner/clinician. It is the insurance provider for the NHS. It provides legal support so that disputes can be resolved in a timely manner and at minimal cost to the organisation. Learning is shared so that risk can be minimised.

More information can be accessed at *https://resolution.nhs.uk/*.

Primary Care Organisations

General and dental practice surgeries, community pharmacies and opticians are all examples of primary care. These provide easy access to help people manage their own health, whether that is by co-ordinating screening programmes, such as the cervical screening programme, or by preventing future problems through regular dental and eye examinations.

Regulatory Bodies

Regulatory bodies oversee registration of many of the professions working within the health and social care sectors. To practise in one of these professions, a person must have completed an approved programme of study and fulfil the relevant regulatory body's requirements for registration. They set standards for professional conduct and education, as well as investigating complaints made about those professionals. The main regulatory bodies associated with medical imaging and radiotherapy staff are as follows:

- the General Medical Council regulates doctors working in the UK;
- the Health and Care Professions Council regulates 15 professions, including radiographers;
- the Nursing and Midwifery Council regulates nurses.

Secondary Care Organisations

If a GP refers a patient on for an expert opinion, then that referral is made to secondary care services, commonly specialty medical practitioners who are based in a hospital setting. The patient may need to attend a hospital or a community hub that provides these services. This care can be planned or elective, but can also be urgent or emergency care.

Tertiary Care Organisations

Tertiary Care Organisations provide highly specialised care and may be within a secondary care setting, for example a specialist Burns Unit. They may also be stand-alone centres of excellence such as a regional oncology or paediatric hospital.

CHAPTER SUMMARY

- Multiple organisations make up the NHS, each with its own unique role in providing health and social care.

- Funding is determined through taxation; it is distributed by the government to the relevant national bodies, and then onwards to the providers.
- Integrated care systems focus on the health and care needs of the local population.
- The Care Quality Commission is the regulator responsible for ensuring that high-quality health and social care is delivered.

REFERENCES

1. The Kings Fund. The NHS Budget and How it has Changed. 2022. Available at www.kingsfund.org.uk/projects/nhs-in-a-nutshell/nhs-budget.
2. NHS England. Integrated Care Systems. Available at www.england.nhs.uk/integratedcare/.
3. Health and Care Act 2022. Available at www.legislation.gov.uk/ukpga/2022/31/contents/enacted.
4. NHS. Transforming Imaging Services in England: A National Strategy for Imaging Networks. 2019. Available at https://webarchive.nationalarchives.gov.uk/ukgwa/20210401201200/https:/improvement.nhs.uk/documents/6119/Transforming_imaging_services.pdf.

SECTION 2

RESOURCE MANAGEMENT – FINANCIAL, HUMAN AND PHYSICAL ASSETS

3. HEALTHCARE BUDGETS

Amanda Martin

INTRODUCTION

Within the healthcare sector, operational service delivery is focused on delivering high-quality timely care to patients within the financial resources available. There is a requirement to deliver services that are said to demonstrate 'value for money', with the objective being to create interlocking services that deliver care focused on health and social needs rather than profitability. Chapter 2 outlines the funding pathway from the UK government to integrated care boards (ICBs) (**Figure 3.1**).

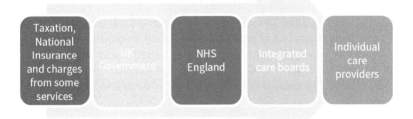

Figure 3.1 Funding process within NHS England.

DOI: 9781003380078-3

This chapter will explore how the funding is transferred to providers and subsequently managed. It is important to differentiate between the terms 'funding' and 'budget'.

- Funding is the money given to the provider by the ICB to carry out the commissioned work in that financial year.
- A budget is the projected cost of carrying out that work. It is defined by the senior leader of the service and the financial team.

PROVIDER FUNDING

Historically, funding for healthcare services in England was governed by the **National Tariff Payment System**, which saw providers being paid based on activity levels. Scotland, Northern Ireland and Wales use block contracts that provide a lump sum of money for a defined service, although there is an element of a tariff scheme within this to determine the cost of the services. A tariff scheme uses set prices for different procedures or treatments that have been agreed nationally based on the average cost of delivering that activity. In England, the National Tariff Payment System was replaced with the **NHS Payment Scheme** (NHSPS) in April 2023; it still uses tariffs, but now referred to as unit prices, to determine the cost of services. This changed the approach to payment for services,[1] with the most relevant changes being:

1. the **aligned payment and incentive approach** (API) for contracts costing more than £0.5M, which combines a fixed payment, a guaranteed amount of income for an agreed amount of activity, with extra payment for any additional activity undertaken.
2. the **block contract**, or lump sum payment, for smaller organisations where activity may be lower and the contract value less than £0.5M.

While pure activity, as in patient numbers, can be recorded, the complexity of care is often not reflected within these numbers. A better demonstration of activity is presented when an episode of care is broken down into a series of codes for procedures and treatments that have taken place, as well as the definitive diagnosis. This is referred to as

clinical coding and is linked to the agreed national prices, informing payments from commissioners. Costs can be associated with individual procedures, but are commonly grouped for Emergency Department (ED), Outpatient and Inpatient attendances, where several procedures may take place within a specific pathway of care. Each individual procedure and associated code can be combined into **Healthcare Resource Groups** (HRGs), groups of procedures commonly carried out in a particular pathway, resulting in one code for that episode of care. Radiology prices are not always included in the HRG, allowing them to be paid for on an individual basis (referred to as unbundled HRGs). Coding is carried out by clinical coders who interpret the clinical information provided at the end of an episode of care and assign the appropriate code. It is complex and requires accurate documentation by clinicians and practitioners of the activity associated with that episode of care. An example of inaccurate documentation can be demonstrated through the recording of a computed tomography (CT) scan attendance. The examination code for a CT scan of the thorax is entered into the radiology information system (RIS) by the administrative staff. The request is vetted, and a decision is made that the patient needs a contrast examination, and it is to include the neck. If the attendance on the RIS is not changed, then the code assigned by the clinical coder will be for a single body part CT scan without contrast, rather than a CT scan of two body parts with contrast. Assigning the correct codes is key to generating the income for the activity undertaken.

Funding from activity is the main source of income, but it can be supplemented by **income-generation schemes**, with additional money often being used to enhance patient care or improve staff experience. The schemes may include the following.

- Food outlets.
- Car parking.
- General over-the-counter medicine sales in the hospital pharmacy.
- Charging for baby scan pictures.
- Joint ventures with optometry companies.
- Offering post-mortem CT imaging services.
- Charging for overseas patients accessing NHS services.
- Treating private patients in NHS facilities. When a private patient attends for diagnostic imaging or therapy, there will be a process

in place for claiming the income, which generally requires the Medical Imaging or Radiotherapy Department to complete forms indicating that the relevant procedure has taken place. Some organisations will distribute private patient funds directly to the relevant departments, where departmental staff can choose how to spend them, for example on continuous professional development (CPD) activities. Other organisations will have a central budget for private patient funding.

- Health Education England (HEE) funding which is generally used for training costs of healthcare professionals.
- Some Medical Illustration services.

For further reading please access:

1. NHS Payment Scheme: *www.england.nhs.uk/pay-syst/ nhs-payment-scheme.*
2. NHS National Tariff Payment System: *www.england.nhs.uk/wp-content/uploads/2020/11/22-23-National-tariff-payment-system.pdf.*

REVENUE AND CAPITAL FUNDING

Funding is allocated to either the revenue budget or a capital budget; one cannot be used to offset the other.

- **Revenue funding** is used for the day-to-day costs of delivering a service, such as staffing costs (pay budget) and consumables (non-pay budget) and is predominantly obtained from the ICB through contracts for commissioned services.
- **Capital funding** is used to purchase an asset that is going to be used for delivering a service in the future, such as the purchase of a new mobile X-ray machine. In the UK NHS, a capital spend is usually an item or a group of inter-related items that costs more than £5,000. It is usual for that asset to be used for more than a period of 1 year following its purchase, with an estimated life expectancy for the asset being issued at the time of purchase (discussed in more detail in Chapter 8). There should be a **capital plan** in place that covers a defined period, for example 5 years, and

includes all items which it is envisaged will be needed during this time. This plan must be reviewed and updated each year. Additional capital funding can be accessed through alternative funding processes that may be available locally, but can also be generated from the sale of assets or donations. A **business case** is needed for a capital spend. This is a structured document that presents the case for investment and includes the following, as a minimum:

- ○ Explanation of the problem that needs to be addressed through additional funding (sometimes referred to as the case for change).
- ○ Option appraisal – the options available for addressing the problem with the preferred option indicated, including the option of doing nothing.
- ○ Costings associated with each option.
- ○ Risks associated with all options, including the option of doing nothing.
- ○ Benefits realisation – the positive outcomes of this investment that may be associated with improvement in delivery of care or financial benefits.
- ○ Stakeholders consulted to ensure that the benefits realised are those required by the stakeholders.

If approved, the funding will become a part of the capital plan and the investment can be made.

BUDGET RESPONSIBILITY

The ultimate responsibility for making sure that the services are delivered within the funding allocated lies with an organisation's **chief executive officer** (CEO), but is managed by the **director of finance**. In collaboration with the financial management team, each divisional/directorate lead, who has delegated **budget holder** responsibility, will agree a cost for delivering their service for the subsequent 12-month period in a process known as budget setting (see below for information on budget setting). They are responsible for the budget performance associated with that service and will oversee income and expenditure.

In addition, their responsibilities include, but are not limited to, the following.

- Balancing the income with the expenditure for both pay and non-pay budgets.
- Ensuring that money is spent only as needed and that the best value for money is achieved.
- Identifying where an overspend may occur and developing a plan to address this so that they remain within budget.
- Approving requests to spend money and to recruit into vacancies. Often recruitment requests need to be signed off by the financial management team in a process called vacancy control. This process will review the reasons for recruitment and determine that all other options have been explored, such as appointing a lower-paid member of staff. It will also ensure that the post lies within the agreed staffing establishment and associated budget.
- Authorising or developing business plans to secure further funding.
- Assessing potential imminent financial risks and raising these with the financial management team, such as key resignations that may require agency spending for backfill.

The budget holder can delegate responsibility for managing a part of their budget to other team members, generally heads of departments or operational business managers, referred to as **budget managers**. They are responsible for ensuring that their own service remains within budget and have similar responsibilities to the budget holder. They may be able to further delegate a smaller element to other team members, such as to a practitioner who has responsibility for a specific element of service delivery; these are referred to as **budget line managers**. An example of this level of delegation is the interventional team lead, who has their own budget allocation for spending on consumables associated with the interventional service. Each person with budget responsibility will be able to approve expenditure to a predefined limit, such as £40,000 for the budget manager and £2,000 for a budget line manager. **Figure 3.2** demonstrates how this delegation may work. Each budget manager is responsible for ensuring that their spending and any income that their service may generate remain in balance. Although the responsibility may have been delegated, the accountability still lies with the budget holder, so this requires some oversight on their part.

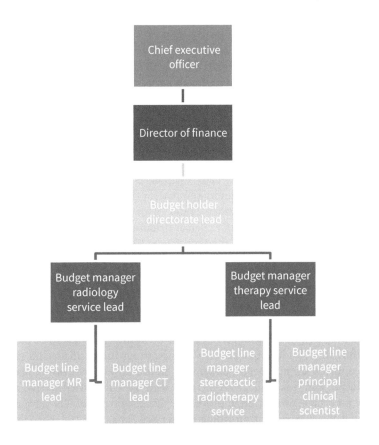

Figure 3.2 Example of budget responsibility delegation.

BUDGET SETTING

Budget setting generally takes place in the months leading up to the next financial year, which commences on 1 April in the UK NHS. It involves the budget holder and the financial management team, with stakeholders such as the commissioners of the service, if relevant, agreeing the amount of money to be allocated to their service and available to spend on delivering that service within a 12-month period. The projected spend for the 12-month period is assessed based on the current service requirements and any future developments. This needs an understanding of **activity trends** and any likely changes year on year, for example an increase in activity for an expensive procedure will require extra funding for both staffing and consumables. Additionally, keeping ahead of **technological developments** is essential so that the budget can be planned according to any new development that may impact on the service within the subsequent 12-month period. This may impact on both revenue budgets for staffing costs and the capital budget for equipment costs. Any foreseeable challenges in workforce recruitment will also need additional funding to pay for the backfilling of vacancies using agency staff, or enhanced rates of pay for substantive or bank staff, which is usually more expensive than the funding released from the vacated post. Indeed, the workforce usually accounts for around 70–80% of the total budget, so it is essential that the budget holder understands the staff costs, as this is key to managing the budget.

As part of budget setting, income-generation schemes may also be discussed. In any department that provides a service, such as radiology, a process of cross-charging allows one department to be paid for the work that they do (income), in preference to being allocated a sum of money within their budget to deliver a service to an unspecified, and often uncontrollable, number of patients. The overall expenditure budget is reduced, and it is reallocated to those who use the service so that they pay for each examination or procedure that they request. The advantage is that the department providing the service is paid for the work that it does; however, if patient attendances fall, the income reduces.

Once the budget is set, there is scope for requesting changes during that budget period for any further unforeseen costs, but it is better, and, in fact, good financial management, to plan the budget in advance to ensure adequate funding is secured for the service that needs to be delivered.

BUDGET STATEMENTS

A budget statement will help manage the financial allocation as it indicates performance against budget and is generally issued monthly for both pay and non-pay budgets. It will identify the **variance**, which is the amount of under- or overspend, with a positive variance representing an underspend and often shown in brackets. There are always risks associated with any budget and early identification of an unexpected overspend will enable further risk to be mitigated by the budget holder and ensure that the annual budget is not overspent. **Budget risk mitigation** is the process of identifying the reason for the overspend and putting plans in place to bring the budget back on track with assistance and advice from the financial management team. An overspend may, for example, be caused by excessive use of bank staff and a review may identify a different way of working that requires less reliance on bank staff. In addition, overspending may also be caused by an increase in use of consumables due to increased activity. This may improve when, and if, the activity reduces, but it may be helpful to seek support from the procurement team to see if it can source a product of similar quality that costs less.

Pay Budgets

Each service will have a **staffing establishment**, an agreed number of staff of each grade that is required to safely deliver the service. The budget will reflect this in **whole-time equivalents** (WTEs), the currency used to record staff costs. This derives from the 37.5-hour working week, as detailed in the terms and conditions of NHS staff,[2] where 37.5 hours equates to 1 WTE. A part-time member of staff is calculated as a percentage of 1 WTE; for example, somebody working 30 hours each week will be 80% of 1 WTE or 0.8 WTE. When staffing costs are calculated, National Insurance and pension contributions are examples of additional costs that need to be considered, commonly referred to as 'oncosts'. This adds approximately 20% to the basic salary. In addition, it is usual to calculate the pay budget based on the midpoint of the pay scale, to allow for staff turnover. If the workforce is static, then the budget should be calculated at the upper end of the pay scale.

The staff budget statement is a list of staff indicating their funded and contracted WTE hours and their hours worked. Each line should be scrutinised to ensure accuracy. **Table 3.1** is a fictional staffing budget statement. It shows us the following:

- Although funded for 1.0 WTE each, Ahmed, Qureshi, Ryan and Young have reduced their hours as indicated in the contracted column; their reductions equate to 1.1 WTE vacancy.

41

- Martyn is contracted for 0.7 WTE but worked 1.0 WTE, meaning that they worked 11.25 hours or 0.3 WTE extra. This will be paid at their standard rate of pay until they have worked more than 37.5 hours, after which they will be paid at the overtime rate.
- The actual requirement for this month exceeds the funded establishment by 0.3 WTE. This may be due to temporary circumstances, such as sickness cover or provision of backlog sessions, or, over an extended period of time, may indicate that the establishment does not match the demand.

The costs will also be calculated for each staff group so that the variance can be identified. **Table 3.2** demonstrates examples of this.

- The funded posts at band 7 are not fully contracted to due to staff reducing their hours. This can change over a year due to individuals' circumstances. This is supported by the underspend seen in brackets.
- There is an underspend at the consultant level associated with 2.1 vacancies.
- Although there are no vacancies at the specialist doctor level (funded posts are contracted to), there is an overspend of £7,206,

Table 3.1 Breakdown of band-7 spend (names are fictitious).

| Band 7 | WTE | | |
	Funded	Contracted	Worked
Ahmed, Z	1.0	0.8	0.8
Downs, E	1.0	1.0	1.0
Humphreys, J	1.0	1.0	1.0
James, A	0.5	0.5	0.5
Martyn, S	0.7	0.7	1.0
Patel, I	0.4	0.4	0.4
Qureshi, U	1.0	0.7	1.0
Ryan, A	1.0	0.8	1.0
Smith, M	1.0	1.0	1.0
Young, J	1.0	0.6	1.2
Total	8.6	7.5	8.9

Table 3.2 Example of excerpt from staffing budget statement.

Staff group	WTE		Year to date (£)		Variance (£)
	Funded	Contracted	Budget	Spend	
Band 7	8.6	7.5	433,440	393,120	(40,320)
Consultant	18.6	16.5	2,507,096	2,224,037	(283,059)
Specialist doctor	1.0	1.0	82,519	89,725	7,206

likely due to extra sessions being provided to accommodate an increase in activity.

■ The overall underspend is £316,173; therefore, this is still within the funded budget.

The budget manager is expected to explain the details of variances through performance meetings within the divisional structure.

Non-pay Budgets

A non-pay budget includes anything that is not directly related to pay. Table 3.3 is a sample fictitious non-pay budget statement; it identifies some of the items that may be included, along with the associated annual budget and year-to-date budget. The expenditure and variance columns enable under- and overspend to be identified.

Table 3.3 Sample fictitious non-pay budget statement.

July 2022	Annual budget	Year to date (£)		
		Budget	Expenditure	Variance
Uniforms	1,603	534	599	65
Stationary	1,406	469	518	49
Contrast	5,104	1,701	1,699	(2)
Drugs	1,202	401	410	9
Dressings	825	275	262	(13)

Numbers in red demonstrate an overspend against the budget.

COST IMPROVEMENT PROGRAMMES

In the UK, the central government sets **efficiency savings targets**, with the target for 2022/23 to 2024/25 being 2.2% each year. This means that the same service must be delivered with 2.2% less money. This efficiency saving is passed down to individual organisations but, in reality, the target set locally is higher as the organisation aims to deliver the service within the funding allocated to them. This local efficiency target is set annually at the start of each financial year and indicates the amount of money, usually presented as a percentage of the budget, that must be saved in that year. A cost improvement programme (CIP) must be developed to deliver on the efficiency target, but still enable safe and efficient care to be delivered.[3] Each department/specialty is given an agreed target of CIP for that year to achieve. This is usually indicated and tracked in their budget statement.

Chapter 10 discusses continuous quality improvement (CQI) as a means of making changes to improve a service. Efficiency savings may be released through CQI, as one of the aims is to eliminate waste; however, the main focus of CQI is on improving the provision of care, whereas the focus of CIPs is to deliver efficiency savings. It is important that a **quality impact assessment** is carried out on any plan that is based purely on saving money to make sure that quality is not adversely affected. CQI and CIPs may run concurrently and may be a part of the same project; however, they can also be carried out independently of each other. Examples of CIPs are better workforce planning and use of skill mix, which releases staffing costs; bulk buying to reduce the cost of consumables; and better use of technology. Savings can take the following forms:

- Recurrent, such as losing a substantive post from the staffing establishment. Unless this post is replaced, the money will be saved every year.
- Non-recurrent, such as the sale of an asset. Selling an asset can take place only once, so the saving can be made within that year only.
- Cash releasing, such as switching to a lower-priced consumable.

- Non-cash releasing, such as increasing the number of CT slots within a session – this increases efficiency as more activity is taking place for the same fixed costs of delivering the session (staffing, equipment, etc.), but direct financial savings are not necessarily made. Non-cash-releasing savings are generally more difficult to quantify as part of a savings target.

Savings cannot be made simply by underspending the budget.

CHAPTER SUMMARY

- There is a need to manage the budget so that services are delivered that demonstrate value for money.
- The majority of income comes from the government through the ICBs, but there are income-generation schemes that an organisation can use to subsidise income.
- Budget setting involves agreeing the budget that is needed/available to be able to deliver the service requirement.
- Revenue funds are used for day-to-day items required for service provision.
- Capital funds are used for large one-off purchases such as equipment and the associated building charges.
- The budget holder can delegate responsibility to a line manager for part of the budget, but accountability for that budget cannot be delegated; it remains with the budget holder.
- The budget statement will help to identify performance against budget and predict any potential overspend on the budget.
- Pay budgets are generated based on the staff within the staffing establishment.
- It is usual for every department to make efficiency savings.

REFERENCES

1. Healthcare Financial Management Association (HFMA). HFMA Introductory Guide to NHS Finance – Chapter 16 https://www.hfma.org.uk/system/files/chapter-16---hfma-introductory-guide-to-nhs-finance.pdf

2. NHS Employers. NHS Terms and Conditions of Service Handbook. 2023. Available at www.nhsemployers.org/publications/tchandbook.
3. HFMA. NHS Finance. 2023. Available at www.hfma.org.uk/system/files?file=hfma-introductory-guide-to-nhs-finance.pdf.

4. WORKFORCE PLANNING

Amanda Martin

INTRODUCTION

Workload across healthcare is increasing for several reasons, including a rise in the ageing population and increased poverty levels, both requiring greater healthcare input. New models of service delivery are being developed to address this increased demand, such as **Community Diagnostic Centres** (CDCs) in England, which aim to deliver faster diagnostic access in the community, away from the acute hospital setting;[1] however, these require additional staff to those already employed in the acute setting. The workforce is already depleted[2,3] for numerous reasons, including:

- a reduction in the number of people coming out of training programmes, which is not meeting the needs of healthcare providers;
- a reduction in the number of posts due to the financial challenges faced by organisations;
- an increase in staff sickness, with mental health illnesses, such as anxiety, depression and stress, being the most common cause of sickness absence;[4]
- an increase in resignations due to the rising workload pressures.

The King's Fund suggests that the challenges have been impacted further in the UK healthcare environment by the lack of workforce planning at government level, although the challenges associated with this are also acknowledged.[5] Workforce planning is not just a government responsibility; it is essential that all managers and leaders are involved

DOI: 9781003380078-4

in local workforce planning for their own services,[6] so that the correct number of staff with the right skills are in the right place at the right time. Robust and inclusive recruitment processes to attract and appoint these staff are needed. In addition, good workforce planning has a positive impact on staff retention as they understand where their role fits in with the organisation and can see future development opportunities that may be available.

WORKFORCE PLANNING

Workforce planning is a means of forecasting and planning workforce needs for the future so that a safe and efficient service can be delivered. This may be short- or medium-term planning for an adaptation of a current pathway mainly impacting on radiology services, or it may be long-term planning for a large project across the wider healthcare economy. The United States Office of Personnel Management (OPM) has identified an uncomplicated way of looking at workforce planning, which is depicted in **Figure 4.1** and outlined in the following sections.[7]

Strategic Planning

Predicting what the future service will look like can be challenging and requires input from key stakeholders from the wider health and social care environment who recognise and understand the needs of the local community and the population that is being served. The organisation's strategic plans, local and national plans and data such as workforce trends should enable a direction to be set for the service to develop that is going to meet those needs. In addition, the Topol review outlines how developments such as artificial intelligence (AI), robotics and digital medicine will change the roles of those who work with this technology, thereby impacting on the skills required.[8] The intentions of those who commission services, emerging health initiatives and technological advancements will inform the workforce plan.

Workforce Analysis

This starts by identifying the roles that will be required to deliver the service, including skills, knowledge and experience of staff involved.

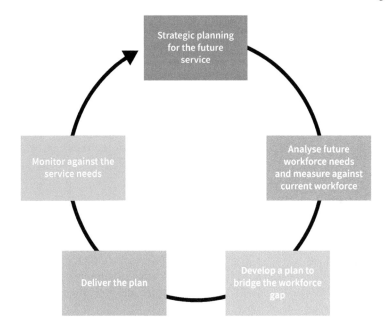

Figure 4.1 Process of workforce planning. (Adapted from OPM.)

This will enable gaps to be identified between the current workforce and the future workforce. Given the significant changes required in diagnostic services,[1] it should not simply be focused on radiographers, but should also explore how other linked professions can contribute to delivering the service, including nursing roles and administrative and clerical staff. This is '**skill mix**' and generally refers to the range of different roles within a team. But this is certainly not new within the UK radiography profession. In 2003, a report was published that outlined the success of skill-mix introduction in breast services by introducing the 'four-tier' model of staffing and recommended that this be rolled out across the remainder of the radiography workforce.[9] Skill mix is key to delivering the workforce requirements of the future and should be used across the whole service delivery, including out-of-hours working. For example, assistant practitioner roles are common in projectional radiography, but less common in cross-sectional imaging.[10] Given the

49

drive for increased capacity within cross-sectional imaging,[1] this is an ideal opportunity to explore the development of modality-specific assistant practitioners.

Although skill mix is used variably across the UK,[11] benchmarking data such as those from the 'Model Hospital' (available at *https://model.nhs.uk*) is useful for informing the workforce plan. Tools are also available to help with identifying the future workforce needs, with the 'Star Model' from Health Education England (HEE)[12] advocating exploring five areas to move forward with workforce redesign, which will inform workforce plans. These are as follows:

1. supply;
2. upskilling (increasing the knowledge and experience);
3. new roles;
4. new ways of working;
5. leadership.

This model has numerous tools and guidance documents to support development of the workforce for the future and is available at *www.hee.nhs.uk/our-work/hee-star*.

Bridge the Staffing Gap

Once the gap in workforce has been identified, then develop an action plan to move forward in bridging that gap and ensure the right people are in the right roles. This may involve upskilling current staff through training programmes, talent management, succession planning and recruitment initiatives to increase staff numbers.

■ **Training programmes** can be focused on all levels of staff and deliver many benefits, not least the demonstration of commitment to staff development. This can include in-house training, for example in cannulation or the use of remote technology for home reporting, or external formal qualifications. In-house training will be essential to address the new models of service delivery and the expected growth within computed tomography (CT) and magnetic resonance imaging (MRI) as there will be a requirement for more radiographers to be fully competent in these modalities.[1] While formal CT and MRI qualifications are available, the speed at which these services are expanding cannot be addressed with formal training alone; delivery of an in-house training programme through rotational posts will be needed. This requirement for increased competence in these areas is reflected in the Health and Care Professions Council (HCPC) Standards of Proficiency.[13]

The formal training route is generally open to registered practitioners, with the aim being to extend their roles into enhanced or advanced practitioner roles and enable existing services to grow, for example radiographer-led gastrointestinal services or reporting services. It also enables new services to be developed, with skills that may have been absent previously now being used in, for example, discharging patients from Emergency Care.[14] These opportunities for career progression will improve recruitment and retention in the workforce registered with the HCPC.

The unregistered workforce is often overlooked for formal training, but their development is key in enabling an appropriate and effective skill mix to support the workforce plan. Referred to as '**grow your own**',[15] developing training opportunities for this cohort of staff will give them job satisfaction and support recruitment and retention, and it is often a cost-effective way to develop and deliver a range of skills focused to local need. Examples of this are in supporting a radiology assistant to become an assistant practitioner or to complete a radiography training programme. Within English NHS organisations, there may be access to apprenticeships that come with funding, referred to as an **apprenticeship levy**, which is often managed through an organisation's education leads.[16] This supports the costs of work-based programmes of study and is available for both unregistered and registered staff. Apprenticeships are especially beneficial for the unregistered workforce as they allow them to continue earning, thereby overcoming the financial barrier that often prevents them from progressing to formal qualification.

■ **Talent management** involves recruiting the right person into the right role, identifying staff members who, with appropriate nurturing and development, can make significant contributions to the service or enabling staff to use their training, education and experience to the best of their abilities, referred to as working to the '**top of their licence**'. It may require different ways of working, often within newly defined roles that extend beyond the traditional uni-professional roles of the past. 'Grow your own' in the registered workforce allows for their development to be supported and for service needs to be met.

■ **Succession planning** involves identifying key positions within the department that are business critical and assessing the skills and knowledge required for those positions. Any staff member who feels that they have the potential to fill that position in the future can then have a development plan to enable them to work towards this.

■ **Recruitment** is possibly one of the most time-consuming elements in delivering the workforce plan as it is unlikely that the plan can be achieved within current staffing levels. Recruitment processes will be discussed in Chapter 5.

Deliver the Actions

Carry out those tasks identified in the action plan to bring the workforce to the required level with the correct skills in place.

Monitor the Plan

Ensure that the actions deliver the needs of the service as identified in the strategic planning stage. If they do not, then adjust the plan. Always be mindful that this is a cyclical process, as the service will always be changing direction as new policies are put in place and demands are made.

CHAPTER SUMMARY

■ Workforce planning is key to ensuring the right staff with the right skills are in the right place at the right time.

■ Analysing future needs requires an understanding of the local population and their health needs, emerging technologies and health initiatives and local and national strategic plans.

- It is essential that skill mix is considered as a means of increasing the workforce.
- The gap between the current and the future workforce can be bridged by training programmes, identifying talent, succession planning and recruitment.

FURTHER READING

- NHS England. HEE Star: Accelerating Workforce Redesign. Available at www.hee.nhs.uk/our-work/hee-star.
- Chartered Institute of Personnel and Development (CIPD). Inclusive Recruitment: Guide for People Professionals. Available at www.cipd.org/uk/knowledge/guides/inclusive-employers.
- NHS Employers. Inspire, Attract and Recruit Toolkit: Resources and Guidance to Support Your Workforce Supply. 2022. Available at www.nhsemployers.org/inspire-attract-and-recruit.
- Health Education England (HEE). What Is Talent Management. 2021. Available at https://library.hee.nhs.uk/learning-academy/talent-management-toolkit.
- NHS England. Workforce Planning and Resource Management. Available at www.england.nhs.uk/mat-transformation/matrons-handbook/workforce-planning-and-resource-management/.
- Society of Radiographers. Return to Practice. Available at www.sor.org/learning-advice/learning/return-to-practice.

REFERENCES

1. Richards, M. Diagnostics: Recovery and Renewal. 2020. Available at www.england.nhs.uk/wp-content/uploads/2020/11/diagnostics-recovery-and-renewal-independent-review-of-diagnostic-services-for-nhs-england-2.pdf.
2. College of Radiographers. *Diagnostic Radiography Workforce 2021 UK Census.* London: Society of Radiographers; 2021.
3. Sloane, C. and Hyde, E. Diagnostic radiography education: time for a radical change? *Imaging and Therapy Practice.* August 2019: 5–10.

4. NHS Digital. NHS Sickness Absence Rates. 2023. Available at https://digital.nhs.uk/data-and-information/publications/statistical/nhs-sickness-absence-rates.

5. Morgan, B. *NHS Staffing Shortages: Why Do Politicians Struggle to Give the NHS the Staff It Needs?* London: The King's Fund; 2022.

6. Department of Health. *A Health Service of All the Talents: Developing the Workforce.* London: Department of Health; 2000.

7. US Office of Personnel Management (OPM). OPM's Workforce Planning Model. Available at www.opm.gov/policy-data-oversight/human-capital-framework/reference-materials/strategic-alignment/workforceplanning.pdf.

8. Topol, E. *The Topol Review: Preparing the Healthcare Workforce to Deliver the Digital Future.* Leeds: Health Education England; 2019.

9. Department of Health Learning and Personal Development Division. *Radiography Skills Mix: A Report on the Four-tier Service Delivery Model.* London: Department of Health; 2003.

10. Snaith, B., Harris, M.A. and Palmer, D. A UK survey exploring the assistant practitioner role across diagnostic imaging: current practice, relationships and challenges to progression. *British Journal of Radiology* 2018;**91**:1091.

11. NHS. *Diagnostic Imaging Network Workforce Guidance.* London: NHS; 2022.

12. NHS England. HEE Star: Accelerating Workforce Redesign. Available at www.hee.nhs.uk/our-work/hee-star.

13. Health and Care Professions Council (HCPC). Standards of Proficiency: Radiographers. 2023. Available at www.hcpc-uk.org/standards/standards-of-proficiency/.

14. Howard, M.L. and Craib, J. Radiographer-led discharge in a minor injuries unit. *Journal of Medical Imaging and Radiation Sciences* 2018;**49**:3.

15. Malhotra, G. *Grow Your Own: Creating Conditions for Sustainable Workforce Development.* London: The King's Fund; 2006.

16. Gov.uk. Pay Apprenticeship Levy. Available at www.gov.uk/guidance/pay-apprenticeship-levy.

5. RECRUITMENT AND RETENTION

Amanda Martin

INTRODUCTION

Whether a vacancy arises due to staff leaving, transferring into training posts, moving into a specialty or through a workforce planning strategy, robust and inclusive recruitment processes to attract and appoint the right staff are needed. The correct practices also need to be in place to retain the staff once in post.

The purpose of the recruitment process is to attract and appoint the most suitable candidate for the post being offered. There are several legislative documents that inform these practices; these will not be covered in detail, but you should be familiar with them:

- Employment Rights Act 1996;
- the Part-time Workers (Prevention of Less Favourable Treatment) Regulations 2000;
- the Fixed-term Employees (Prevention of Less Favourable Treatment) Regulations 2002;
- Equality Act 2010;
- Data Protection Act 2018.

Recruitment practices are not purely focused on the legal requirements and the ability of the candidate to answer the questions or complete the tasks that have been set. From developing the **job description** (JD) and **person specification** (PS) to advertising and interviewing, inclusive practices must be embedded to eliminate bias or discrimination and

DOI: 9781003380078-5

ensure that all potential applicants have an equal opportunity to be successful regardless of their socioeconomic background or protected characteristics. The Chartered Institute of Personnel and Development (CIPD) offers a comprehensive guide to inclusive recruitment (*www. cipd.org/uk/knowledge/guides/inclusive-employers*).

CONTRACT TYPES

On appointment, the employee will be given a written state-ment of particulars in the form of a contract, which outlines the terms and conditions of employment, including rights, duties and responsibilities. The contract type will depend on the job advertised and offered.

- *Full-time* – the maximum number of weekly hours for that post must be worked. This is defined as 1 whole-time equivalent (WTE) and is currently 37.5 hours in the NHS.
- *Part-time* – a percentage of the maximum number of weekly hours is worked. This is usually defined in hours and as a part of the WTE; for example, if 1 WTE is 37.5 hours, then 0.8 WTE is 30 hours. The terms of employment will be the same as for a full-time staff member, but the number of days paid annual leave will be pro rata, based on the maximum numbers of days paid annual leave for the individual's years of service.
- *Fixed term* – this is often referred to as a temporary contract and is for a defined period. The terms of employment will be the same as for a permanent member of staff and the hours worked may be full-time or part-time.
- *Annualised hours* – a fixed number of hours are worked over a 12-month period, but these are not distributed equally across the year. The hours may be distributed so that the employee does not work school holidays, for example, and the total number of hours worked each week may vary, but the pay will be evenly distributed across the 12-month period. This allows for flexibility for somebody with carer responsibilities.
- *Bank* – also called a zero-hour contract. The staff member works only when asked to work.

- *Agency* – this is generally negotiated with an individual agency with an agreed time frame and pay scale for the duties requiring cover. The government has rules for use of agency staff in the NHS,[1] which outline the maximum fee that can be paid per hour for an agency worker.
- *Secondment* – this occurs when a staff member is transferred to another role for a defined period, but is expected to return to their own role at the end of the contract. These allow staff to develop skills that they may not necessarily be exposed to in their substantive role. The terms and conditions of their own role remain throughout the secondment.

THE RECRUITMENT PROCESS

The recruitment process takes time and is costly, so it is essential to ensure that good practices are followed, from the first indication that a vacancy may arise through to appointment of the successful candidate. Attracting, appointing and retaining the right candidate is key to a stable and happy workforce.

The Job Description and Person Specification

When a vacancy arises, it is wise to review the JD to make sure that it accurately reflects what the department needs. It is easy to simply recruit 'like for like', but a vacancy may be an opportunity for change and to add different abilities and expertise to the department. The JD is an essential part of the recruitment process as it is a summary of the most important aspects of the role, and all applications will be measured against this. It also allows the potential candidate to get an understanding of what the job entails. Alongside the JD, there must be a PS. This defines the competencies and behaviours required for the role; the criteria must be objective and measurable. It includes the **essential criteria** to be able to carry out the role, such as educational qualifications, experiences, skills and abilities. There may also be **desirable criteria**, those elements that would be nice but are not essential, and these are useful in shortlisting if the post attracts a lot of applications. Most organisations will have a template for completion of these two documents.

Advertising a Vacancy

Marketing a vacancy is essential to attract candidates. There are many student placement sites: developing a sense of belonging within the student on placement is likely to influence them to seek employment with the organisation.[2] Open evenings, study days and bespoke student placements will introduce the organisation to other potential candidates and enable them to get a feel for the hospital and department. In addition, working with and maintaining high visibility in local educational institutes will demonstrate the commitment that the department has to educational development. Recruitment fairs also allow an organisation to market itself and attract a greater number of applications by raising its profile.

Part of the **marketing strategy** is the development of an **advert** that immediately draws the attention of a potential candidate. This will be the first opportunity to make an impression, so it is important to sell your organisation, department and post, but to maintain an honest approach and not offer anything that will not be achievable, as this will affect retention. It is also essential to consider the words used in the advert, in order to not introduce bias in, for example, age or gender. It is good to start with some broad statements about the organisation and then focus down to the specifics of the role. Use keywords, taken from the JD, against which you can measure applications; for example, if you indicate that you are a student placement site, then you would expect applicants to outline their experiences in supporting others in the workplace. Decide on where the post will be advertised, for example will it be an internal recruitment process, or is there a need to search from a wider pool of potential applicants? There may be a **talent pool** within the organisation. This is generated if a recent recruitment drive resulted in good candidates not being offered a post due to lack of vacancies. Any candidates in this pool who meet the criteria for the post can be invited for an informal discussion and offered the post without advertising or interviewing again. They usually remain in the talent pool for a limited period of time, usually around 6 months, after which they will have to reapply for any subsequent vacancies. If external recruitment is chosen, then consider using social media to promote the vacancy. Advertising vacancies in the NHS is generally done on the NHS Jobs platform (*www.jobs.nhs.uk*), but it may be possible to define where the advert needs to be displayed, such as within specific journals or on certain websites where those suitable for the job may be particularly active. Groundwork done prior to the recruitment cycle will greatly assist in attracting enough applicants from which to select the best candidate.

Shortlisting the Applicants

Some recruitment software packages allow filter questions to be used that may reject some applications based on pre-set requirements. Once the advert has closed, all applications passing this first filter stage must be reviewed in a process called **shortlisting**, the purpose of which is to identify those candidates to be invited to interview. The application must be measured against the JD and PS so that objectivity is maintained. It is good practice for two people to do this; ideally, one of these will also be on the interview panel. This stage of the process is the reason that care must be taken in writing the JD and PS. For example, if you are looking for somebody with skills in student support, you will not be able to exclude a candidate who does not mention this unless you have specified it in the JD and PS. Candidate applications that meet the essential criteria should be invited to interview; however, if this is a large number, then it may be necessary to use the desirable criteria as the deciding factor. Candidate applications that do not meet the essential criteria must be rejected, with reasons indicated to ensure openness and transparency. Carelessness in writing the JD and PS may result in the best candidate being rejected and the appointed candidate struggling to fulfil your needs.

The Interview Stage

The interview invitation must outline any assessment that will be part of the interview process. A practical-based simulation, for example, will allow some soft skills, such as patient/practitioner interaction, to be measured, while an image viewing test may give a good indication of technical standard, both of which are difficult to measure on application and through **interview questions**. Prior to interview, develop a scoring mechanism based on what the best candidate would look like. Again, this introduces some level of objectivity and removes the subjectivity, bias or discrimination that can sometimes arise. Candidates with pro-tected characteristics as outlined in the Equality Act 2010[3] must be given the same opportunity as other candidates. Those with a disability may require adjustments, but this should not detract from a good can-didate being appointed.

Interview questions must be developed that allow the interviewers to determine whether the candidate is motivated and able to do the job for which they are being interviewed. This is their opportunity to demonstrate that they fulfil the requirements as outlined in the JD and PS, often by expanding on the content in their application. The same questions must be asked of all candidates. However, the inter-viewers can probe a little deeper into statements made in the applica-tion process, for example a candidate may indicate that they have been involved in research or audit. It is acceptable for the interviewer to seek further detail on this despite research/audit not being a defined inter-view question. A scoring mechanism for the interview questions will be useful in differentiating between different candidates.

Figure 5.1 demonstrates the process of recruiting the successful can-didate, from development of the JD to interviewing for the single cri-terion of student support. It is recognised that students who are being interviewed for their first post may not necessarily have experience in supporting other students, unless within a mentor role; therefore, the essential criterion is evidence of supporting others. This may be evi-denced through their experience at school/college or in a part-time job.

Once the successful candidate has been selected, **pre-employment checks** will be carried out by the Human Resource (HR) department, such as checks of identity, professional registration and qualification, as well as references, safeguarding and health. The successful candidate must be informed that any offer is subject to these checks being com-pleted successfully.

International Recruitment

An individual from abroad can apply for any advertised role and must be considered alongside all other applications. If appointed, they may require a work visa and processes must be followed to ensure the cor-rect visa is acquired. While this is recruiting from abroad, it is not the

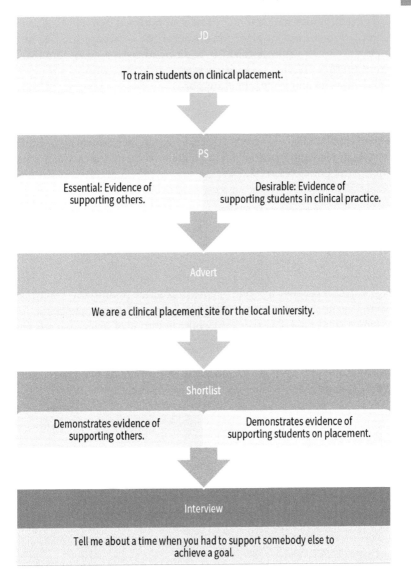

Figure 5.1 Recruitment process for the single criterion of student support.

full extent of international recruitment as outlined by NHS England.[4] There are processes in place for organisations to secure funding and support to recruit from abroad.[5] In addition, there is guidance for managing the new recruit's transition into a different culture, with personal, pastoral and professional support.

Recruitment Agencies

There is an abundance of agencies that can support recruitment both within the country and internationally. They will find the candidates who fit your criteria and arrange interviews at a convenient time for both employer and employee. There is a significant fee associated with this service.

Return to Practice

A previously registered radiographer who has been out of the workplace for several years may wish to return to practice; this can be successful in a supportive environment. The returnee must develop their own learning plan and complete a period of clinical practice prior to becoming registered again. This can be done on a formal contract of employment, for example being paid at a lower level while the period of supervised retraining takes place, or on an honorary or volunteer contract. The contract must specify the process following the application for re-registration, for example appointment into a substantive post or termination of the contract depending on the outcome of the application.

RETENTION STRATEGIES

Once appointed, a good retention strategy is key to ensuring staff longevity and that staff stay in post. NHS England states that retention is a key priority across the NHS[6] through valuing, supporting, developing and investing in people; this can be done through several schemes.

Induction

Induction is the first encounter that a new starter will have with the workplace; it is the organisation's opportunity to make a good impression, as this period of their employment is one that they are likely to remember for a long time. Dedicated orientation and socialisation time is important to allow the new starter to adjust to their new working environment. Research suggests that a lack of support in this regard negatively impacts retention.[7] It is likely that the organisation has a corporate induction package that aims to introduce the new starter to the organisation, but each department also needs an induction package focused on their own area. An **induction package** may have different elements depending on the job role and experience of the individual, so it should be adaptable in its design. As a minimum, an induction package must include the following:

- a tour of the workplace, identifying fire escapes and crash trolleys, and introducing key staff members;
- reminder of crash call and fire procedures, which is also likely to be covered in the corporate induction days;
- a discussion about relevant HR practices such as sickness reporting and booking annual leave;
- an introduction to rostering and how to manage shift requests, if this is relevant;
- training on any software systems and medical devices;
- location of all policies and procedures and reading of those relevant to the role;
- continuous professional development opportunities available;
- check of practical aspects such as car parking, identification (ID) badges, intranet access, uniform ordering, locker provision and information about any coffee scheme;
- a list of all mandatory and statutory training requirements and those local competencies that must be achieved before a practitioner is able to work as an independent practitioner.

It can also include the practical elements associated with the role and within the JD, an outline of the probationary and preceptorship period, if relevant, and a discussion about expectations on both sides. Remember that this initial period in post can be overwhelming, and it is important to recognise when a new starter is possibly drowning in information overload. A change of direction may be needed, and this may be the chance to get them to work alongside somebody who is already doing the job. This will refocus them so that when they return to the induction, they know why they are doing it.

Probation

Most employees have a probationary period during which a new starter will need to meet certain expectations around attendance, attitude, behaviours and clinical skills, for example. This period generally lasts for 6 months, and it enables the new starter to gain an understanding of their new role while providing the leader with a framework for assessing the performance of the new starter and, through a series of meetings, addressing any concerns early enough in their employment to be impactful. The new starter should, through the recruitment and induction processes, understand what their new role entails, but expectations should be reiterated at the commencement of employment and at the start of the probationary period. If, through regular review meetings, it is identified that these expectations are not being met, then supportive mechanisms need to be put in place. This is also an opportunity for 'checking in' with the staff member to see how they feel that they are progressing, particularly if they are not in a preceptorship programme. At the end of the 6-month period, the leader decides whether to continue to a permanent contract for the new starter, terminate the contract due to failure to complete relevant competencies or extend the probationary period if it is felt that there is the possibility that competencies will be achieved imminently. Although this can be seen negatively by the new starter, in that they can be dismissed if they do not meet expectations, it should be presented as a supportive mechanism to ensure that the possibility of termination is minimised for those who do not meet expectations at the outset of their appointment. Should termination be inevitable, HR must be involved, and the organisation processes followed.

Probation runs alongside preceptorship for clinical staff members, and part of the probationary expectations will be that good progress is being made with their preceptorship competencies.

Preceptorship

The Department of Health (2010)[8] defined preceptorship as:

> *a period of structured transition for the newly registered practitioner during which he or she will be supported by a preceptor to develop their confidence as an autonomous professional, refine skills, values and behaviours and to continue on their journey of lifelong learning.*

A structured and practitioner-centred preceptorship programme focuses on the transition from supervised student to accountable and autonomous practitioner, and is a unique opportunity to demonstrate, at an early stage in the appointment, commitment to staff development. It has been demonstrated that the lack of such a programme negatively impacts staff retention.[9] This phase in a newly registered practitioner's career is pivotal to their own development, but also to their understanding of the accepted values and behaviours of the organisation. It is central in allowing them to develop confidence by consolidating their academic knowledge and applying it to their new role through supernumerary and independent clinical practice, but also to experience professional socialisation beyond that which they were exposed to as a student.[10,11]

A comprehensive preceptorship programme is necessary to ensure equity in access and to minimise variation in levels of support for all newly qualified practitioners. Many models have been proposed, mainly for the nursing profession, with very few directly related to radiography.[8,12,13] There is not one model that can be applied to all situations; however, there is a commonality in all models. They all advocate a supportive approach, with a named **preceptor** who must be a role model demonstrating the expected standards and behaviours of the organisation. The preceptor needs excellent technical skills, but also the ability and confidence to give constructive feedback and discuss areas for improvement to facilitate reflection and learning. Although they may not necessarily work alongside the practitioner in clinical practice, they play a pivotal role in supporting their integration into the established team and in helping them to take responsibility for their own learning. That said, the preceptor should work with the new starter in the first week. A close relationship between the preceptor and practitioner at this early stage is mutually beneficial as it supports growth for the practitioner in a safe environment and allows an element of job satisfaction for the preceptor as they facilitate that growth.[14] Meetings with the preceptor can then be weekly, encouraging the practitioner to reflect on their practice over the past week and addressing any areas of concern so that escalation does not develop into loss of confidence. Preceptor training does take place in many organisations, and it may be useful to identify experienced staff who have an interest in this role and in accessing this training prior to newly registered practitioners commencing in post.

Any preceptorship programme must be built around the needs of the role to which the practitioner is being appointed. For example, there will be an expectation that a newly qualified radiographer fulfils certain criteria within the first 6 months of commencing in post. These may be related to undertaking all general radiography examinations, working in theatre and performing basic computed tomography (CT) scans so that they can be rostered safely to out-of-hours shifts. The programme must enable fair rotation through these areas, initially in a **supernumerary** capacity, but then working independently. If supernumerary practice cannot be supported, it is recommended that the practitioner works near experienced staff so that they can easily seek guidance if needed.

Although there is some element of structure to this approach, with rostering through specific areas within the workplace to ensure all aspects of the role are covered, there must be flexibility to accommodate for the different rates of development among different practitioners. A defined set of **competencies** for each area will enable the preceptor to see if the practitioner is at the required level for safe autonomous practice in that area and will also allow the practitioner to reflect on those areas that may need a little extra time. Competencies must be based on the key aspects of the role and aligned with the JD, for example safe use of equipment, radiation protection and the demonstration of an understanding of fundamental departmental protocols and procedures.

As the practitioner completes the formal period of the preceptorship programme, it is important to maintain that preceptor support over the subsequent months with ad hoc meetings driven by the practitioner. This will prepare them for their first appraisal where, hopefully, there will be a noticeable change from nervous new starter to accountable and professional practitioner, demonstrating effective practice with the appropriate attitudes and behaviours required of a healthcare professional.

Appraisal

Appraisal is undertaken annually, with key review dates set within the intervening months; it is an essential process in demonstrating commitment to staff development. It should be carried out by somebody who has been trained in undertaking appraisals; most organisations offer in-house training. There are two parts to the appraisal conversation:

1. Provide assurance that the staff member is carrying out their role as expected through review of the previous 12 months, discussion of any challenges and achievements, and assessment of evidence demonstrating progress against previous performance objectives.
2. Support the staff member to work to the top of their licence and to achieve their career aspirations by looking forward to the next 12 months and identifying the support needed for the next step on their career pathway through the setting of performance objectives and production of a new **personal development plan** (PDP). This can be used as part of their ongoing re-registration portfolio.

Specific, measurable, achievable, relevant and time-bound (SMART) objectives must be set each year and aligned with the organisational goals. In addition to assisting in securing any required funding for training programmes, this also enables the individual to see how their role directly impacts the organisation. The PDP will assist in meeting these objectives by outlining any learning or development activities needed, but may also include activities that support personal growth, such as shadowing a senior staff member or experiencing work in another area.

The appraisal is an opportunity to formally recognise the contributions of a staff member and should be positive, supportive and confidential. The staff member should be encouraged to talk openly about their past experiences and future desires and the appraiser should use both verbal and non-verbal communication styles that demonstrate a real interest. When discussing areas for improvement, constructive feedback should be given. If a staff member is the subject of formal performance management, this should be acknowledged, but this is not a time for performance management discussions as these should already be being managed appropriately. If a staff member is performing particularly well, then a talent conversation can be included in the appraisal. This enables a specific development plan to be agreed that is focused on fast-tracking them into a specific role.

CHAPTER SUMMARY

- Successful recruitment relies on good marketing strategies and a clear JD and PS to match candidates against.
- Inclusive recruitment practices are essential to avoid bias and discrimination.
- Recruitment can also be achieved through agencies, international recruitment and by attracting practitioners back into the workplace with a package of support.
- Retention of staff requires focused support through induction, probationary and preceptorship packages.
- Appraisals give a staff member the time to reflect on their current role, discuss career aspirations and explore present or future suitable opportunities. It also contributes to succession planning.

REFERENCES

1. Gov.uk. Rules for all Agency Staff Working in the NHS. 2015. Available at https://www.england.nhs.uk/wp-content/uploads/2023/04/Agency-rules-changes-for-2024-to-2025.pdf.
2. NHS England. Reducing Pre-registration Attrition and Improving Retention. Available at www.hee.nhs.uk/our-work/reducing-pre-registration-attrition-improving-retention.
3. Equality Act 2010. Available at www.legislation.gov.uk/ukpga/2010/15/contents.
4. NHS Employers. International Recruitment Toolkit. Available at www.nhsemployers.org/publications/international-recruitment-toolkit.
5. Mulshaw, C. *Allied Health Professions: Quick Guide to International Recruitment.* Leeds: Health Education England; 2021.
6. NHS England. Looking after Our People – Retention Hub. Available at www.england.nhs.uk/looking-after-our-people/.
7. NHS England. Using Induction to Support Retention. Available at www.england.nhs.uk/nursingmidwifery/healthcare-support-worker-programme/attracting-people-into-healthcare-support-worker-roles/using-induction-to-support-retention/.

8. Department of Health. Preceptorship Framework for Newly Registered Nurses, Midwives and Allied Health Professionals. 2010. Available at www.cntw.nhs.uk/wp-content/uploads/2017/09/NTWC22-App1Precepframework-RCN-V02.pdf.

9. Cox, D. Good preceptorship positively impacts staff recruitment and retention. *Nursing Times* 2022. www.nursingtimes.net/opinion/good-preceptorship-positively-impacts-staff-recruitment-and-reten-tion-02-02-2022/.

10. Strudwick, R., Mackay, S. and Hicks, S. Cracking up? The use of dark humour in the radiography department. *Synergy* 2012;4–7.

11. Strudwick, R.M. Keeping it professional. *Imaging and Therapy Practice* 2014;26–30.

12. Nisbet, H. A model for preceptorship – The rationale for a formal, structured program developed for newly qualified radiotherapy radiographers. *Radiography* 2008;**14**(1):52–56.

13. Martin, A. and Dodd, E. First steps into practice: The value of preceptorship. *Imaging and Oncology* 2020;34–39.

14. Harvey-Lloyd, J. and Morris, J. Supporting newly qualified diagnostic radiographers: Are we getting it right? *International Journal of Practice-based Learning in Health and Social Care* 2020;**2**:57–67.

6. STAFF ENGAGEMENT

Louise Kemp

INTRODUCTION

> *The performance of any healthcare system ultimately depends on its people – the NHS is no exception.*[1]

Chapter 5 outlined the importance of good recruitment and retention practices to ensure that the correct person is appointed and remains in post. Links between staff retention, reduction in agency and bank spend, and employee engagement are recognised.[2] NHS England describes these engagement strategies as actions that make staff feel valued and supported and allow them to develop in order to achieve their potential.[3] This is demonstrated in the Healthcare Leadership Model dimension 'engaging the team', defined as 'Involving individuals and demonstrating that their contributions and ideas are valued and important for delivering outcomes and continuous improvements to the service'. Crucially, this dimension also describes lack of engagement as 'building plans without consultation, autocratic leadership, failing to value diversity and springing ideas on others without discussion'.[4]

There are many and varied definitions of staff (or employee) engagement, although it is often described in terms of a 'psychological state', with overarching themes around levels of employee connection to an organisation and commitment to organisational goals. One definition is:

> *… a workplace approach resulting in the right conditions for all members of an organisation to give of their best each day, committed to their organisation's goals and values, motivated to contribute to organisational success, with an enhanced sense of their own wellbeing.*[5]

                                          DOI: 9781003380078-6

It is important to be able to express what staff engagement is to be able to measure how engaged the workforce is. Engaged staff are fulfilled within their role, show lower sickness absence rates, lower staff turnover and reduced absenteeism (being off work without good reason).[6] They are more likely to deliver high-quality care and to think creatively.

FUNDAMENTALS OF ENGAGEMENT

To be engaged, a staff member needs to have their basic needs met. They need to have support for their health and wellbeing, a sense of belonging and to feel accepted, encouragement and recognition of their achievements and an environment in which to flourish. This principle, Maslow's hierarchy of needs, is applied to all aspects of life[7,8] and can be adapted to address staff engagement (**Figure 6.1**). If basic needs are met, a staff member is likely to be satisfied in their role. There is a relationship between job satisfaction and staff engagement. Just as a low level of job satisfaction can lead to lack of engagement, a lack of engagement can impact on job satisfaction.

Staff engagement requires an understanding of staff expectations to ensure that they, as well as staff needs, are met. The NHS People Promise,[9] developed as part of the NHS People Plan,[10] which aims to make the NHS the best place to work, identifies behaviours expected of senior staff and colleagues (**Figure 6.2**). These leadership behaviours should reflect the organisational values, one of the four key enablers for employee engagement,[11] with the others being:

■ provision of strong strategic narrative and a shared vision;
■ empowerment of staff who are treated with respect;
■ seeking out and listening to employee voices.

Regular staff surveys are an effective barometer of how engaged staff are feeling. The findings can aid development of targeted engagement activities and initiatives and allow the effectiveness of the improvements to be measured. In addition, the NHS conduct national quarterly and annual surveys. The annual survey provides

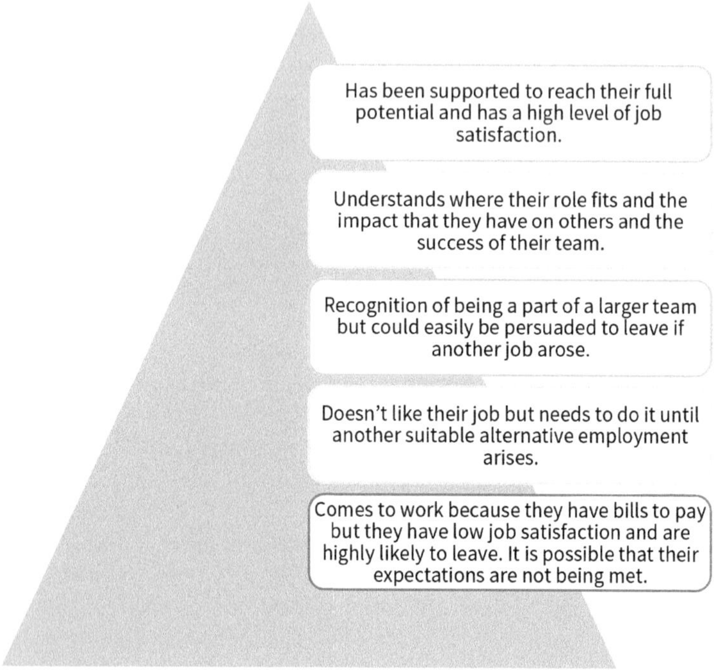

Has been supported to reach their full potential and has a high level of job satisfaction.

Understands where their role fits and the impact that they have on others and the success of their team.

Recognition of being a part of a larger team but could easily be persuaded to leave if another job arose.

Doesn't like their job but needs to do it until another suitable alternative employment arises.

Comes to work because they have bills to pay but they have low job satisfaction and are highly likely to leave. It is possible that their expectations are not being met.

Figure 6.1 Maslow's hierarchy of needs, adapted for staff engagement and retention.

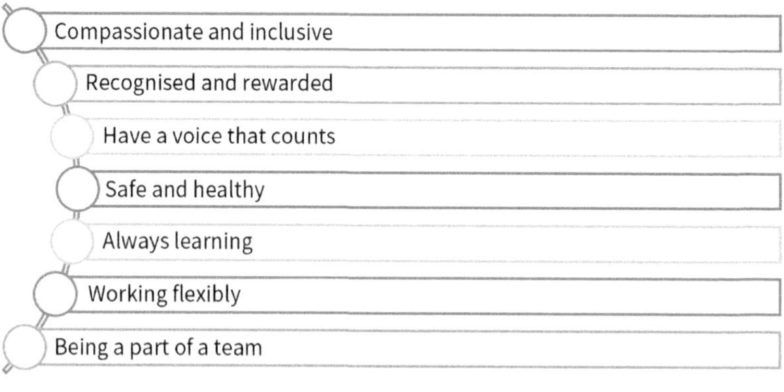

Compassionate and inclusive

Recognised and rewarded

Have a voice that counts

Safe and healthy

Always learning

Working flexibly

Being a part of a team

Figure 6.2 The NHS People Promise.

official data on employee experience across organisations, enabling benchmarking of performance in different measures at local and national levels. The quarterly survey allows more frequent analysis of engagement with individual organisations. Alternative sources of information such as sickness absence, turnover rates, appraisal feedback or face-to-face 'check-ins' can be indicative of how successful staff engagement is.

PROMOTING HEALTH
AND WELLBEING

Engagement is linked to health and wellbeing.[12] Positive action to promote health and wellbeing can improve satisfaction and engagement. The words 'health' and 'wellbeing' are often used together, but what do they mean?

- *Health*: the constitution of the World Health Organization (WHO) describes health as being: 'a state of complete physical, mental and social wellbeing and not merely the absence of disease or infirmity'.[13]
- *Wellbeing* is defined as 'how people feel and how they function, both on a personal and a social level, and how they evaluate their lives as a whole'.[14]

It is clear that wellbeing goes beyond a state of good health and incorporates a sense of satisfaction with all aspects of life.

Good-quality data can help in analysing health and wellbeing themes; a dashboard will allow themes, trends and gaps to be demonstrated, and the effectiveness of interventions to be identified. Data may originate from:

- existing sources of data:
  - NHS surveys;
  - electronic staff records;
  - audits of sickness/absence to identify areas of concern;
  - exit interviews;
- data arising from identified gaps in information:

73

- targeted surveys;
- listening events.

The data may be quantitative, such as sickness/absence rates, staff turnover or incident reporting, or qualitative, from appraisals, exit interviews or complaints. Providing a variety of channels to solicit feedback on staff health and wellbeing, such as surveys, drop-in sessions or suggestion boxes, will assist in retrieving a broad range of data from which proactive preventative strategies and action plans can be produced. It is important to follow up staff feedback with action to give staff confidence that engagement is genuine and meaningful.

In 2017, the National Institute for Health and Care Excellence (NICE) published a quality standard in relation to employee mental and physical health and wellbeing (**Figure 6.3**).[15] This was followed

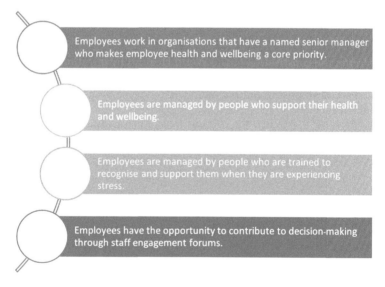

Figure 6.3 Adapted from the NICE quality standard for mental health and wellbeing. (© NICE. 2017. QS147: Healthy workplaces: improving employee mental and physical health and wellbeing. Available from www.nice.org.uk/guidance/qs147. All rights reserved. Subject to Notice of rights. NICE guidance is prepared for the National Health Service in England. All NICE guidance is subject to regular review and may be updated or withdrawn. NICE accepts no responsibility for the use of its content in this product/publication.)

in 2021 by the NHS Health and Wellbeing Framework,[16] which built on the NICE standards by recognising that health and wellbeing is not purely focused on physical and mental health, but also incorporates other factors impacting on the ability of an employee to bring their best self to work. These are as follows:

- improving personal health and wellbeing;
- relationships;
- fulfilment at work;
- managers and leaders;
- environment;
- professional wellbeing support.

Improving Personal Health and Wellbeing

Physical and mental/emotional health are not mutually exclusive; a healthy lifestyle, incorporating diet, exercise, sleep, hydration and managing smoking, drugs and alcohol consumption, can contribute to improvements in both. A healthy lifestyle is an important element of both day-to-day wellbeing and longer-term disease prevention. However, data show that mental health illnesses were consistently the most reported reason for sickness absence in 11 out of 12 months of 2022, a trend that continued into 2023, with 20-25% of those off sick citing mental health illness as a reason.[17] Poor mental health is usually associated with anxiety, depression and stress, but may also be linked to financial distress or menopause symptoms. The NHS provides a range of supportive mechanisms to address issues that may impact on mental health, for example the promotion of discount schemes and assistance with childcare costs to support improved financial management. Additionally, the NHS has recognised the negative impact that the menopause could have on a workforce in which over 75% of employees are female,[18] and advocates the development of a supportive environment to positively impact the health and wellbeing of these staff members and improve retention. Other supportive measures may include the following:

- providing access to organisational resources and employee assistance programmes;
- offering targeted interventions such as physiotherapy support;

- upskilling staff to help improve their own health and wellbeing and that of others;
- implementing measures to manage and reduce stress, such as workload management strategies or mindfulness sessions;
- ensuring staff can take sufficient rest and breaks from work, including taking annual leave;
- facilitating access to physical activity during the working day, for example encouraging staff in office-based roles to get up and move about regularly or provision of on-site gym facilities;
- completing risk assessments for vulnerable staff and making adjustments to help them manage their health at work.

Relationships

Staff are entitled to be treated with dignity and respect at work. The quality of relationships can have a huge impact on how staff feel about coming in to work. Positive supportive relationships within teams creates a sense of unity and belonging and improves team working. Supportive measures may include the following:

- regular wellbeing conversations;
- developing forums to encourage peer support;
- creating opportunities for shared activities;
- providing training to staff in giving and receiving feedback;
- providing staff with the skills and confidence to speak out when they witness negative behaviours.

Fulfilment at Work

Fulfilment at work is described in a number of ways:[16]

- bringing your whole self to work;
- achieving work–life balance;
- carrying out a role that offers purpose, potential and recognition.

It is more than just the day-to-day work. It brings together different elements that contribute to personal health and wellbeing, both physical and mental. Supportive measures may include the following:

- actively promoting and facilitating equality and diversity, for example timing meetings and events to ensure cultural and religious inclusion;

- flexible working policies and rostering, designing roles to offer flexible working by default;
- ensuring staff have access to mentoring, coaching and career development;
- ensuring workloads are manageable;
- making sure staff take their annual leave;
- recognition of the positive contribution of staff;
- ensuring job roles are enriching and fulfilling.

Managers and Leaders

The behaviour of leaders has a direct impact on those around them. A compassionate and inclusive culture depends on compassionate and inclusive leaders. These behaviours are enshrined within a values-based leadership culture in which the leader is able to communicate a common set of values, build alignment through recognition of each team member's values and strengths, and subsequently develop trust within the team. Supportive measures may include the following:

- encouraging autonomy within teams;
- communicating effectively;
- involving staff in decision-making and service improvement;
- aligning policy and practice to organisational and employee needs;
- upskilling managers in how to have health and wellbeing conversations;
- providing clear expectations by setting goals and objectives;
- helping staff to see the value of their role;
- creating psychological safety, thereby ensuring staff can have honest conversations with managers and feel able to speak out if they have concerns;
- keeping an eye on presenteeism (working longer hours than required) and leavism (catching up on work during leave).

Environment

Many Medical Imaging and Radiotherapy Departments were planned and built decades ago, creating limitations in existing departmental layouts. This does not mean they cannot be safe, clean and comfortable, with safe spaces for staff to rest and recover. New builds should be designed with ergonomics in mind. The term 'environment' may also describe how a department feels culturally. The workplace should be a healthy and supportive environment with an open and inclusive culture. Supportive measures may include the following:

- ensuring a safe working environment with appropriate personal protective equipment (PPE) and effective infection prevention and control procedures;
- applying zero tolerance to bullying, harassment and abuse;
- giving access to green space;
- promoting a culture of psychological safety and mental wellbeing where staff feel able to openly discuss mental health and seek/ receive help;
- ensuring staff feel safe to, and know how to, raise concerns, with access to 'freedom to speak up' guardians within the department.

Professional Wellbeing Support

Organisational support is available from the Occupational Health Department, Human Resources, the Chaplaincy Service and via access to other specialist knowledge agencies. Some organisations form partnerships with employee assistance programmes; leaders should be aware of the help available to be able to appropriately signpost staff. Supportive measures may include the following:

- training departmental health and wellbeing champions;
- dedicated 'health and wellbeing' notice boards or areas to promote available resources;
- mental health first aiders.

ENGAGEMENT ACTIVITIES

While promoting health and wellbeing, it is also important to consider engagement activities. Although there are likely to be many initiatives offered at organisational level, such as 'benefit and reward' schemes and staff networks, departmental leaders are key to local-level staff engagement and developing a compassionate and inclusive culture within a team. Visible leadership support is key for staff engagement to be successful; staff engagement should be part of the quality and governance agenda and data should be used to monitor trends. Examples of actions and initiatives to improve engagement include the following:

- **Respecting and valuing diversity:**
  - consideration of the timing of meetings and events to respect religious practices, for example Friday prayers, to ensure these are inclusive;
  - celebrating cultures and groups such as LGBTQ+ Pride;
- **Recognising contributions:**
  - helping staff to feel valued by acknowledging effort and saying thank you;
  - celebrating successes both inside and outside the workplace;
  - 'Going the Extra Mile' awards/initiatives;
  - mechanisms to facilitate peer-to-peer recognition;
- **Communication:**
  - providing clear, timely and accessible information to employees and their representatives via social media, staff forums or newsletters;
  - engaging in coaching and mentoring activities;
- **Giving staff a voice:**
  - holding listening events;
  - including staff in service improvement activities;
- **Staff development:**
  - upskilling, coaching and mentoring;
  - appraisals;
  - providing continuing professional development (CPD) opportunities;
- **Retention:**
  - 'itchy feet' or 'stay' conversations with staff at risk of leaving, or planning to leave, the organisation;
  - talent management activities to motivate staff to stay.

COACHING AND MENTORING

Teaching, mentoring and coaching are important components in staff engagement as they enable regular communication and support and motivate staff to achieve their potential. The experience and skills of staff will determine where they sit on the coaching continuum (**Figure 6.4**), and they will likely benefit from supervision in the early days of their career. These supportive mechanisms are for everyone, not just those experiencing difficulties, and can be beneficial to both parties, the coachee and the coach, with the additional benefits of improving performance and communication, and reducing staff turnover.

Restorative supervision, an element of the Advocating for Education and QUality ImProvement (A-EQUIP) model,[19] adopted in midwifery and nursing from 2017, has not yet been formally adopted within the Allied Health Professions, but this practice is transferable and worth considering. It is concerned with creating space and time for staff to slow down and be able to engage in discussion and reflection, while receiving 'supportive challenge and open and honest feed-back'. Within the nursing profession, this is a practice supported by professional nurse advocates – clinical leaders who support nursing staff to develop personally and professionally.

Mentoring is the sharing of knowledge, skills and experience, with a focus on professional development and growth. It is directive and comes from the perspective of the mentor, who is usually more experienced/senior and works in a similar field. The mentoring relationship is long term, with a focus on career and personal development, encouraging autonomy and building confidence. Mentoring is not the same as line management; instead, it is about creating a safe space for the mentee to talk and learn, with an emphasis on the needs of the individual.

Coaching is the use of questioning and listening skills to help an individual achieve personal and professional success by prompting them to reflect on their experiences and come to their own conclusions on the best course of action. Coaching is non-directive and comes from the experience of the individual being coached. It is 'non-hierarchical' and does not require professional expertise or skills in the field of the coachee. Coaching tends to be shorter term, with a focus on particular issues or development needs. National training programmes in coaching are available from numerous sources including the NHS Leadership Academy.

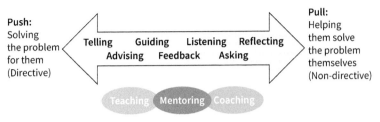

Figure 6.4 The coaching continuum.

Coaching Conversations

Coaching conversations differ from coaching sessions as they tend to be more spontaneous. They should be positive and supportive, with an emphasis on asking rather than telling. Having an effective coaching conversation does not require any training and is dependent on using these active listening skills:

- paying attention and being present;
- being curious and asking open-ended questions: *'What are your thoughts on ...?' 'Tell me about ...'*;
- allowing the person time to think and respond; being comfortable with silence;
- checking your understanding by reflecting and summarising what the person has said: *'It sounds like you're saying that ...'*;
- withholding judgement and advice;
- summarising the key themes and next steps.

Coaching Models

There are many coaching models; however, the GROW model is perhaps the most well-known.[20] GROW stands for:

- *Goals* – identify the end point and the goal to be achieved;
- *Reality* – determine the current position and available opportunities;
- *Options* – identify the options available and any barriers to be overcome;
- *Will* – identify the next steps for achieving the goals.

CHAPTER SUMMARY

- Retention and engagement are linked.
- Engaged staff are more likely to deliver high-quality care and have job satisfaction.
- To be engaged, a staff member needs to have their basic needs met.
- Staff engagement requires an understanding of staff expectations to ensure that they, as well as staff needs, are met.
- Engagement is dependent on the health and wellbeing of the staff member.
- Positive action must be taken to promote health and wellbeing in order to improve satisfaction and staff engagement.
- Supportive mechanisms must be in place to enable staff to bring their best self to work.
- Appropriate activities will allow increased engagement.
- Teaching, mentoring and coaching are important components in staff engagement as they enable regular communication and support and motivate staff to achieve their potential.

FURTHER READING

- NHS England. Looking after Your Team's Health and Wellbeing Guide. Available at www.england.nhs.uk/long-read/looking -after-your-teams-health-and-wellbeing-guide/.
- NHS Leadership Academy. Healthcare Leadership Model. Available at www.leadershipacademy.nhs.uk/healthcare-leadership-model/.
- Chartered Institute of Personnel and Development (CIPD). Employee Engagement: Definitions, Measures and Outcomes. 2021. Available at www.cipd.co.uk/Images/employee-engagement-discussion-report _tcm18-89598.pdf.
- Bailey, C., Madden, A., Alfes, K., Fletcher, L., Robinson, D., Holmes, J., et al. Evaluating the evidence on employee engagement and its potential benefits to NHS staff: A narrative synthesis of the literature. *Health Services and Delivery Research* 2015;3(26).

REFERENCES

1. NHS England. *The NHS Long Term Plan*. Leeds: NHS England; 2019.
2. Dawson, J. and West, M. *Employee Engagement, Sickness Absence and Agency Spend in NHS Trusts*. London: The King's Fund; 2018.
3. NHS. Looking after Our People – Retention Hub. Available at www.england.nhs.uk/looking-after-our-people/.
4. NHS Leadership Academy. Healthcare Leadership Model. Available at www.leadershipacademy.nhs.uk/healthcare-leadership-model/.
5. CIPD. Employee Engagement: Definitions, Measures and Outcomes. 2021. Available at www.cipd.co.uk/Images/employee-engagement-discussion-report_tcm18-89598.pdf.
6. The King's Fund. *Staff Engagement: Six Building Blocks for Harnessing the Creativity and Enthusiasm of NHS Staff*. London: The King's Fund; 2015.
7. Maslow, A. A theory of human motivation. *Psychological Review* 1943;**50**(4):370–396.
8. Institute for Healthcare Improvement (IHI). *Framework for Improving Joy in Work*. Boston, MA: IHI; 2017.
9. NHS England. Our NHS People Promise. Available at www.england.nhs.uk/our-nhs-people/online-version/lfaop/our-nhs-people-promise/.
10. NHS England. We Are the NHS: People Plan for 2020/21 – Action for Us All. Available at www.england.nhs.uk/publication/we-are-the-nhs-people-plan-for-2020-21-action-for-us-all/.
11. MacLeod, D. and Clarke, N. *Engaging for Success: Enhancing Performance through Employee Engagement*. London: Office of Public Sector Information; 2009.
12. Cartwright, W. (chair). Sustaining Employee Engagement and Performance: Why Wellbeing Matters. 2012. Available at https://engageforsuccess.org/wellbeing/sustaining-employee-engagement-and-performance/.
13. WHO. Constitution of the World Health Organisation. 1946. Available at https://apps.who.int/gb/bd/pdf_files/BD_49th-en.pdf#page=6.
14. New Economics Foundation. *Measuring Wellbeing: A Guide for Practitioners*. London: New Economics Foundation; 2012.

15. NICE. Quality Standard [QS147]. *Healthy Workplaces: Improving Employee Mental and Physical Health and Wellbeing.* Available at www.nice.org.uk/guidance/qs147.
16. NHS England. *NHS Health and Wellbeing Framework.* Leeds: NHS England; 2021.
17. NHS Digital. NHS Sickness Absence Rates. 2023. Available at https://digital.nhs.uk/data-and-information/publications/statistical/nhs-sickness-absence-rates.
18. NHS England. *Supporting Our NHS People through Menopause: Guidance for Line Managers and Colleagues.* Leeds: NHS England; 2022.
19. NHS England. A-EQUIP Model: A Model of Clinical Midwifery Supervision. Available at www.england.nhs.uk/wp-content/uploads/2017/04/a-equip-midwifery-supervision-model.pdf.
20. Whitmore, J. *Coaching for Performance: GROWing Human Potential and Purpose: The Principles and Practice of Coaching and Leadership.* London: Nicholas Brealey Publishing; 1992.

7. MANAGING ATTENDANCE AND POOR PERFORMANCE

Amanda Martin

INTRODUCTION

Chapter 4 outlined the purpose of workforce planning and the need to identify the correct roles with the associated knowledge and skills required to deliver the service, based on the demand and complexity of the service, but also considering any learners working in that area. As such, there is likely to be a diverse workforce undertaking different tasks and working at different levels. Appropriate management of this workforce is needed so that safety and efficiency are maintained. At a fundamental level, this involves the following:

- having a fair and equitable rostering system that considers safe staffing numbers and skill mix;
- managing annual leave (AL) so that safe staffing levels are always maintained;
- managing sickness absence to minimise disruption caused by unplanned fluctuations in staffing levels;
- managing poor performance or behaviours that may compromise safety and efficiency.

Some management processes, such as capability and disciplinary management, as well as the later stages of attendance management, can be distressing and complex procedures; the Human Resource (HR) department will be available for support. HR departments have a range of policies that should be consulted to inform the leader on what should be

DOI: 9781003380078-7

done in a particular situation. An HR advisor will advise leaders on the application of those policies and support them through the processes.

Staff being managed on these pathways should be encouraged to seek support; this may be from a colleague, where appropriate within the process, or through union representation, if they are a union member. The role of a union is to represent its members and to protect their rights in the workplace, as well as to provide guidance and support to the staff member throughout the process. It will make sure that policies are being applied fairly and it will be the link between the staff member and the HR department.

ROSTER MANAGEMENT

Rosters should be produced that are fair and equitable to all staff, considering staffing numbers and skill mix needed to ensure safe practice. **Electronic rostering** software packages are available and there is an expectation that they will be used by those working in the NHS to assist in getting the right balance between patient safety, efficiency and cost.[1] In addition to producing rosters, electronic rostering allows for:

- management of AL;
- management of sick leave;
- management of other leave, for example carers leave and maternity leave;
- management of time in lieu (TL);
- access to data associated with, for example, appropriate staffing levels and equity of shift distribution.

The data associated with the rosters can be easily accessed and used in workforce management reviews. Such packages may also be useful outside the public sector, depending on the staffing numbers involved.

Roster development can be time-consuming, despite electronic rostering automating the process. It is beneficial to have a roster co-ordinator who has oversight of roster production. In addition, there may be a small team of staff members who have also been trained on the use of the rostering software and can help with roster production, approval of AL and making the daily roster changes that are inevitable, such as sickness recording.

A roster is likely to encompass all locations within a department, indicating shifts to be covered, minimum staffing numbers and the required skill mix. If there are numerous shifts to cover across a 24-hour period, then all staff must be rostered equally through all shifts, ensuring good rotation between different areas so that skills are maintained. There are occasions when a staff member may have been advised by the Occupational Health (OH) department to not work shifts for health reasons; this would have been conveyed to the leader in the OH report following an ill health referral. Additionally, a staff member may have an agreement in place to work a set shift pattern that suits their personal needs, referred to as a '**flexible working agreement**'. The roster team should be familiar with these variations and ensure staff are appropriately rostered.

It may be useful to commence roster production by rostering available staff to those locations or shifts where staffing numbers are crucial to the ability to deliver the service. This will leave the less crucial locations/shifts uncovered if there are periods of high vacancy or staff absence rates. A decision can then be made about whether to cover these shifts or not. Staff must not be rostered extra hours to ensure that all locations/shifts are covered. **Working time regulations**[2] suggest a maximum number of hours to be worked each week. Exemptions include 24-hour services and emergency services; however, it is good practice to make sure that staff do not work excessive hours and have appropriate weekly rest periods. There are several options available for dealing with shortfalls in staffing numbers, most of which will need the permission of the person with budget responsibility.

■ Asking substantive staff to work **overtime** ensures that the correct people with knowledge of the workplace are delivering the service, but also overburdens them, with some potentially working a dangerous number of hours. In addition, overtime payments can become expensive if many shifts need covering.
■ Some departments may be able to offer **TL** of hours worked. However, this time needs to be taken at a later date, which may be difficult and cause additional problems if staffing challenges are long term.
■ **Bank** and/or **agency** staff can take the pressure off substantive staff, although care needs to be taken if substantive staff also work

on the bank. The advantage of bank staff over agency staff is that they are generally familiar with the workplace and the costs are lower, but both options can leave the workplace vulnerable if staff decide not to attend at the last minute. Agency staff do tend to take a longer contract so there is some security in long-term cover, but the costs are higher.

- The use of an **on-call system** will provide flexibility, as staff are called in only when needed, but this is generally used outside normal working hours. A staff member being called in overnight may impact on staffing levels the following day, so this needs to be considered when planning the roster.

A **shift leader** must be identified on the roster so that everybody knows who the responsible person is at all times of the day and night. They will be responsible for managing the roster daily, planning staff deployment in response to sickness and workload pressures, and approving TL requests, for example.

Once the roster has been produced, it should be published at least 6 weeks in advance of the roster start date.[3] This leaves time to secure cover for uncovered shifts, as well as allowing staff time to plan their personal life around their allocated shifts.

ATTENDANCE MANAGEMENT

It is essential that there is oversight of staff attendance in the workplace and that absence from the department is correctly managed, whether that is AL or sickness absence. There are other forms of absence, such as study leave, bereavement leave and leave for looking after dependants who are ill, in addition to maternity/paternity/adoption leave, but undoubtedly the biggest challenge to any department is uncontrolled AL and unplanned absence due to sickness.

Managing Annual Leave

To manage any service effectively and efficiently, it is essential that the correct number of staff are in work to deliver that service. An AL agreement will enable some control over the number of staff unavailable to work. There is likely to be an organisation-wide policy that will define a maximum percentage of staff to be on AL at any one time; this will be included in the staffing establishment (the number of posts required to maintain a service). Identifying how that equates to actual numbers of staff will determine the available AL slots each day. It is important to not go above this number, but it is just as important to not be too far below this number. Regularly having too few staff on AL will result in the inability to accommodate everybody's AL in the leave year. In addition, it is essential that staff take their AL entitlement for their own health and wellbeing. While some organisations do allow unused AL days to be transferred to the next leave year, others don't, so those days will be lost. Alongside the organisation-wide policy, it is useful to have a **local agreement** addressing the processes for requesting and approving AL. The following are some points for consideration:

- Identify maximum AL by grade/skill mix so that it does not impact on any one aspect of service delivery.
- Indicate the time frame for requesting AL, for example AL cannot be requested less than 6 weeks before the leave dates.
- Outline special arrangements for dealing with requests for popular holiday times. Consider looking back at AL in previous years for the same period, so that the same staff do not regularly have the same popular holidays approved.
- Identify whose responsibility it is to ensure that cover is provided for shifts vacated due to late AL requests being approved. Beware of this being one person's responsibility as it can be a very onerous task, especially if late AL is regularly approved.

Managing Sickness Absence

The approach to managing sickness absence should always be support- ive and reasons for the absence should not be doubted, but it is essential that all episodes of sickness are managed appropriately, fairly and con- sistently. Future absences may be averted or reduced if a staff member is supported to return safely to their workplace. In addition, it may be possible to manage some episodes of illness while remaining in the workplace with appropriate support.

Managing staff who have been absent due to illness can be an uncom- fortable experience for some. There is the perception that this is a neg- ative, and sometimes punitive, process, but it can have positive benefits for the staff member if the correct process is followed and appropriate support mechanisms are used.

Staff must be encouraged to contact the department at the start of their sickness period indicating how long they feel that they may be absent so that any shortfall in staffing can be addressed. In the public sector in the UK, any sickness absence of less than 7 days requires self-certification, with a formal sickness certificate being required after 7 days' absence.[4] Absences are classified as **short term**, usually less than 4 weeks, and **long term**, usually more than 4 weeks. Short-term absences are managed on the whole when the staff member returns to the workplace, whereas long-term absences are managed while the staff member is still absent. Whether the sickness absence is short or long term, on return to the workplace it is good practice to have an informal return-to-work meeting with the staff member to discuss the reason for absence and identify any support that can be put in place, such as referral to OH. OH focuses on the health and wellbeing of staff in the workplace. While they do not deal with any medical conditions that the staff member may have, they will assess the impact that the condition has on their ability to carry out their role and make recommendations to ensure their health and wellbeing is managed appropriately.

Each workplace will have its own policy for managing frequent short-term sickness episodes or periods of long-term sickness, but it is common to have **thresholds**, or **triggers**, at which review meetings will commence.[3] These triggers will indicate when a review meeting takes place, based on:

- a number of days or episodes of sickness in a defined time period;
- an identified pattern of sickness, for example having the same period of absence off each year.

If, during the **return-to-work** meeting, it is identified that a trigger has been reached, the staff member must be invited to a review meeting so that the episodes of sickness and support offered can be reviewed and further support put in place to help the staff member to maintain their attendance. A **monitoring period** will be defined, and the staff member will be expected to maintain their attendance at work during this period. If they fail to do so, or continually re-trigger outside the monitoring period, they are likely to progress through a defined number of stages, with the final stage potentially resulting in termination of employment.

A staff member who is on long-term sick leave is likely to reach a trigger if triggers are based on the number of days of absence; however, this trigger is not usually managed until they return to the workplace. Instead, a series of meetings should be held at regular intervals throughout their sickness absence, aimed at supporting them to return to work safely. It is good practice to refer any staff member on long-term sick leave to OH for guidance on managing their illness when they return, such as adaptations to either their workplace or roster.

Some staff members will not be able to return to their normal role and **redeployment** must be explored if they can continue to work in another role, or **ill health retirement** if it is not felt that they will be able to work in the foreseeable future. If they can return to work, then monitoring will take place for reaching a trigger, as previously outlined. At all long-term sickness absence meetings, the staff member should be invited to bring a colleague or union representative for support, often referred to as the companion. While both are there for emotional support, they will also be allowed to speak on behalf of the staff member, for example to present their case. However, they may not be allowed to answer questions on behalf of the staff member, although some employers may agree to this.

Special circumstances surround staff members with a disability, and these must be addressed in an organisation's policy for managing sickness. The Equality Act 2010[5] requires reasonable adjustments to be made to enable a disabled person to work, and this may involve adjustments to sickness monitoring and triggers. For example, absences related to their disability may be excluded from the trigger system. In addition, pregnancy-related sickness is generally excluded from any trigger system.

MANAGING POOR PERFORMANCE

On appointment, each staff member receives a contract setting out employment conditions, responsibilities and duties. In addition, they have a job description setting out expectations of them within their role, and some may have standards set by professional/regulatory bodies.

Everybody should be supported to meet these standards, using practices outlined in Chapter 6. However, if a staff member fails to meet the required standards, often identified through an incident or complaint, or by direct observation of poor working practices, this needs to be managed appropriately. The effects of poor performance are widespread: colleagues become frustrated, patient care can suffer and complaints and incidents may increase. Swift action is required to prevent escalation. The initial approach is **informal**, aimed at identifying any difficulties the staff member may have and supporting them to improve their practice. There are numerous reasons for poor performance.

- *Health related*: if the cause of poor performance is **health related**, appropriate referral to the OH service must be considered. They will be able to advise on any required changes to the job role and an expected time frame for resolution.
- *Personal problems*: if poor performance is not health related, but is due to **personal problems**, there are many staff support systems in place. These may differ between organisations, but the OH service and HR advisors should be able to advise on these.
- *Lack of skills or knowledge*: occasionally, a staff member may not have the skills or knowledge to undertake a task that is expected of them. In this instance, a **capability management** process will support them to become competent and capable of undertaking the required task.
- *Poor attitude to work*: rarely, a staff member may demonstrate poor performance due to a poor attitude to their work. They may be appropriately skilled and have the knowledge to carry out their role, but knowingly fail to meet the required standard or to improve on poor performance that has been previously identified and discussed with them. This requires **disciplinary management**.

Although the initial approach should be informal, a staff member can be placed on immediate formal monitoring if a patient has been harmed because of their inability to carry out any aspect of their role or if their poor performance breaches a disciplinary rule. A review of **fitness to practice** and referral to the relevant health regulator may also be necessary, depending on the circumstances.

Capability Management

If it has been identified that the staff member does not have the skills or knowledge to carry out their role to the required standard, then a capability management process should be followed. The first **informal** meeting is normally led by the direct supervisor, such as the team leader. It should result in an action plan being agreed with objectives that will help the staff member to achieve the required level of performance in a specified time frame (**Table 7.1**). Depending on the impact of poor performance on the staff member, the team, the service and the patient, a shorter time frame may be beneficial to minimise risk. It may be useful for the staff member to identify a colleague with the relevant skills and attitude who is willing to support them in achieving these objectives. Regular **review meetings** will enable progress to be assessed and, if at the end of the specified time frame, performance has improved, then the process of review should stop, but it may be beneficial to continue with the peer support.

Informal communication styles can be used at this stage with, for example, an email summarising each review meeting. Retaining a copy of any communication in the staff member's personal file enables this to be referred to if any future capability concerns are raised, but is generally referred to only if further concerns are raised within 2 years.

If performance does not improve, the review period may be extended. This is useful if significant progression has been made and it is felt that the staff member can achieve the objectives if given a little more time.

Table 7.1 Example of an action plan.

Expected level of performance	Gap identified	Objective	Action	Support	Timescale
Diagnostic images to be produced when imaging children	Lack of experience in imaging children	To have confidence in producing diagnostic images of all children	Work alongside colleague with extensive paediatric experience	Roster planning required; colleague to deliver practical guidance	4 weeks

93

If progression has been minimal, then extending the review period is unlikely to result in the desired aim. A more **formal** process of review must then be considered.

It is usual for the person conducting the informal review to refer this on to a more senior staff member who will also involve the HR department. The role of the HR advisor is to advise on the organisational policies and procedures, and to ensure that the correct and fair process is being followed. Together they will conduct the first formal meeting. It is useful, at this point, to review the action plan and outcomes from the informal process. The action plan may be enhanced with educational input or dedicated time for further professional development activities to support progress. A formal letter sent to the staff member should document the ongoing poor performance, reiterate the required level of performance and state the objectives that they must meet. The performance of the staff member should again be reviewed over a defined period of time, during which regular documented meetings will help to determine progress and identify where additional support may be needed. At the end of this period, a decision must be made about onward management.

- Where improvement can be demonstrated, with the required objectives having been met, this should result in the capability monitoring being stopped. However, continued peer support may be beneficial.
- If concerns remain and objectives have not been met, then the process may be continued, particularly if some progress has been made. Each further review meeting must be clearly documented with progress towards meeting the objectives and new time frames for achieving this.
- If it is apparent that the staff member is not capable of carrying out their role despite interventions, and continued review may impact negatively on all involved, then it is usual for a more senior staff member to progress to the next stage, which may involve **redeployment or termination of contract**. If suitable alternative employment is available, this must be considered depending on the nature of the poor performance. This could be a move into a different job role or downgrading and taking on less responsibility. If suitable alternative employment is not available, then a contract can be terminated.

Disciplinary Management

There are times when a staff member might demonstrate a poor attitude to work that manifests as poor performance or inappropriate behaviours. They likely understand the required standard, but knowingly fail to meet it; in this instance, disciplinary management is required. Offences are classified as **misconduct** or **gross misconduct** (**Table 7.2**). These offences are generally referred to as disciplinary rules, and breaking these rules may ultimately lead to dismissal. Good process is essential and those involved in disciplinary action should act fairly and consistently. Disciplinary processes can be stressful and time-consuming and all efforts should be made to conduct the process in a timely and efficient way. Organisations may offer training on conducting disciplinaries, and it may be beneficial to seek out a mentor for support and guidance if inexperienced at conducting these.

If it is suspected that a disciplinary rule has been broken, the first step is to undertake a **fact-finding exercise** to identify the facts associated with the alleged offence, unless the facts are obvious and undisputable. This should be conducted swiftly, usually by the team leader, through interviewing witnesses and gathering evidence, which will then

Table 7.2 Examples of disciplinary rules.

Misconduct	Gross misconduct
Unauthorised absence including continued lateness for shifts	False information given in application for the role
Failure to follow policies or procedures	Alcohol or drug use affecting performance
Verbal abuse	Working elsewhere while off sick
Unjustified refusal to carry out a task	Theft from or fraud against the organisation
Acts that could cause harm to a patient or colleague	Wilful harm to a patient, or to a colleague or member of the public while on duty, including bullying and harassment
Breach in regulations not causing harm	Sleeping while on duty
	Breach of confidentiality

inform the next step. It is important to interview the staff member under investigation first so that they can present their response to the allegation. They must be informed of the purpose of the fact-finding exercise and told not to discuss this with anybody else. They can be accompanied by a colleague who can give pastoral support but will not be able to answer questions. Alternatively, a trade union representative will be able to present the response on behalf of the staff member, act in an advisory capacity and ensure that due process is followed, but they cannot normally answer questions on their behalf. An HR advisor does not need to be involved at this stage, but they should be informed that a fact-finding exercise has commenced, as it may progress to a disciplinary investigation. If the staff member chooses to be accompanied by their union representative, it may be beneficial to invite the HR advisor for mutual support.

Others may be invited for interview based on the discussion with the staff member or based on other pieces of evidence such as work rosters, patient records or, depending on the focus of the investigation, social media posts. When conducting interviews, it is useful to consider the focus of concern and write the questions prior to the interviews. Detailed notes should be made and signed as being an accurate representation of the discussion. Once interviews have been completed and evidence collected, the facts are usually presented to a senior staff member who will consult with the HR advisor and determine the next step. If it is decided that a disciplinary rule has been breached, then a disciplinary investigation will be commissioned. In some instances, usually involving significant breaches of the disciplinary rules, the fact-finding stage may be omitted, and it will go straight to a disciplinary investigation. HR will identify an **investigating officer**, usually somebody outside the staff member's own department, to carry out an independent unbiased investigation within terms defined by the organisation's disciplinary rules, for example in relation to time frames in which the investigation is to take place.

It is essential that the investigating officer meets with the staff member as early as possible and informs them of the reason for the investigation, indicating which disciplinary rule they have allegedly breached. Depending on the risk associated with the potential offence, a staff member may be able to continue in their normal role while the investigation takes place. However, it may be necessary to remove them from their normal workplace if patient safety is felt to be at risk. **Suspension** is not always necessary and should be avoided if possible as it has a negative connotation. It can adversely affect the mental health of the staff member[6] and is seen as a form of punishment. **Redeployment** to a non-patient-facing role may be possible, and it is advisable to have a discussion with other areas to see if they can support the staff member while the investigation takes place.

The investigating officer must review the fact-finding evidence. Further questions may arise from this and they may want to re-interview key witnesses. If a fact-finding exercise has not taken place, the investigating officer will conduct this. At the conclusion of the investigation, they will produce a report, which will be submitted to the HR advisor and the person commissioning the disciplinary investigation. A decision will be made.

- No evidence that a disciplinary rule has been breached.
- There has been a minor misconduct, but a disciplinary rule has not been breached. In this case, it is usual for an informal meeting to take place with the staff member, outlining the behaviours requiring change, the support offered and the target date for improvement. This can be conducted by their team lead. Regular documented review meetings will allow progress to be monitored.
- A disciplinary rule has been breached and a disciplinary hearing is needed. This is a formal process used to determine the outcome for the staff member. During this hearing, the investigating officer will be required to present the report to a panel comprising an independent member of the senior leadership team and a senior HR advisor. It is usual for the report to be shared with the staff member so that they can plan for the hearing with their support colleague or trade union representative, who can be present throughout the hearing. Although it may be found that there is, in fact, no case to answer, this is less likely at this stage. The outcome of the hearing is dependent on the severity of the offence.
  - First written warnings are issued if the offence is a minor misconduct.
  - Final written warnings are issued when a first written warning has been issued but there has been no improvement. The staff member may be removed from

their role and redeployed to an alternative location or into a lower-paid role. This is generally termed 'action short of dismissal'.

○ A combination of first and final written warning may be issued in cases of a serious nature that do not warrant immediate dismissal, but a repeat of the behaviour is unacceptable.

○ Dismissal can take place without issuing a warning if the offence is gross misconduct or if a final warning is in place and action has not been taken by the staff member to make improvements. Dismissal must take place only when there is undisputed evidence against the staff member.

In all cases, it is important to clearly outline the disciplinary rules breached and the behaviours that contributed to this. Expected improvements should be clearly stated and the consequences of no improvement on future management outlined. The length of time that the warning will remain on the staff member's record must be indicated. Every staff member has the right to appeal a decision that has been made that has resulted in disciplinary action; this process should be explained in the letter sent to the staff member. An appeal is generally heard by a different member of the senior leadership team than the one who conducted the hearing.

CHAPTER SUMMARY

- Managing attendance is essential in ensuring safe service delivery for both staff and patient.
- Attendance management includes co-ordination of leave, including AL and study leave, as well as managing sickness absence.
- Sickness absence management should always be supportive and consistent across all staff members.
- Rosters can be complex when multiple shifts are required to cover a service, but use of a rostering team will ensure timely production of rosters that are fair and equitable.
- Managing poor performance can be stressful for all involved, but it should commence with an informal approach before progressing to a more formal process.

- Disciplinary management may be required if a staff member demonstrates poor performance or poor behaviour, and a formal process should be followed, commencing with a fact-finding exercise to determine if a disciplinary offence has been breached. Only once this has been completed should a disciplinary procedure commence.
- All meetings must be documented, either formally or informally, and kept within the personnel file of the staff member.

FURTHER READING

- NHS. Flexible Working in the NHS – A Toolkit for Individuals. Available at www.england.nhs.uk/wp-content/uploads/2022/06/flexible-working-toolkit-for-individuals.pdf.
- Gov.uk. Flexible Working. Available at www.gov.uk/flexible-working/applying-for-flexible-working.

REFERENCES

1. NHS England and NHS Improvement. E-rostering the Clinical Workforce. 2020. Available at www.england.nhs.uk/wp-content/uploads/2020/09/e-rostering-guidance.pdf.
2. The Working Time Regulations 1998. Available at www.legislation.gov.uk/uksi/1998/1833/contents.
3. Carter, P.R. Operational Productivity and Performance in English NHS Acute Hospitals: Unwarranted Variation. 2016. Available at https://assets.publishing.service.gov.uk/media/5a80bdfae5274a2e87dbb8f5/Operational_productivity_A.pdf.
4. Gov.uk. Taking Sick Leave. Available at www.gov.uk/taking-sick-leave.
5. Equality Act 2010. Available at www.legislation.gov.uk/ukpga/2010/15/section/5.
6. Acas. Suspension during a Work Investigation: Supporting Mental Health. Available at www.acas.org.uk/suspension-during-an-investigation/supporting-an-employees-mental-health.

8. ASSET MANAGEMENT AND PROCUREMENT

Amanda Martin and Philip Webster

INTRODUCTION

An asset is defined as:

> *something valuable belonging to a person or company that can be used for the payment of debts.*[1]

All assets are listed on an asset register; this may be devolved down to departmental level for management purposes. The highest-value assets in a Medical Imaging or Radiotherapy Department are the machines (**Figure 8.1**), so this chapter will focus on the procurement and the management of such equipment, but first it will introduce the purpose of asset management.

ASSET MANAGEMENT

Assets are managed through the maintenance of an asset register, a list of capital assets made up of equipment and buildings owned by the organisation and, within the UK public sector, costing more than £5,000. This limit was set by the Department of Health and Social Care (DHSC) as a capitalisation threshold. **Capitalisation** is a method used by accountants to recognise depreciation by spreading the cost over the lifespan of the asset. The threshold of £5,000 can be for a

DOI: 9781003380078-8

single item or for a group of items that individually cost more than £250 and are interdependent, known as grouped assets.

Every asset will have a unique number allocated to it by the organisation – the **asset identification number** – and it is this number that identifies it on the organisation's **asset register**. The register lists all assets owned by the organisation and must include comprehensive information in relation to all assets, including those within the Medical Imaging or Radiotherapy Department. The following are examples of items that may be found on an asset register:

- imaging equipment;
- linear accelerators;
- contrast injectors;
- computers;
- image display monitors;
- patient trolleys and chairs;
- drugs fridge.

Management of these assets is done through a local asset register, extracted from the organisational asset register. This is owned by the manager or senior leader within the department responsible for the use and maintenance of these assets.

It may be beneficial to have a separate asset register specifically for radiology or radiotherapy equipment, separating these items from other assets, such as patient trolleys or computers, for example. This allows clear visibility of the status of all the equipment as it brings together information in one place, allowing for real-time data, which can be used to develop a replacement cycle for the equipment. Such a register must include the following, as a minimum:

- Description of equipment with model number.*
- Name of manufacturer.*
- Unique equipment identifier – serial number.* In addition, there will be a number allocated from the organisation's asset database and printed on the associated asset identification label.
- Location of equipment.
- Year of manufacture.*
- Procurement date.

- Procurement route – direct purchase, managed equipment funding, donation, transfer from another department.
- Value – to include costs such as maintenance charges and capital costs.
- Date of purchase.
- Installation date.*
- Life expectancy.

* These items are identified in the UK Ionising Radiation (Medical Exposure) Regulations 2017 (IRMER), which requires an up-to-date inventory of equipment for compliance.[2]

All radiology and radiotherapy equipment has a lifespan after which the equipment deteriorates leading to increased breakdowns, decreased image quality and the potential for an increase in radiation dose to staff and patients. According to the European Society of Radiology (ESR) and the European Coordination Committee of the Radiological, Electromedical and Healthcare IT Industry (COCIR), the lifespan of both diagnostic and therapy equipment is 10 years, and they recommend that every department has a 5-year forward plan covering any likely equipment replacements, which should be reviewed annually.[3,4] Regular replacement of equipment will improve patient safety, as newer equipment normally gives a lower radiation dose and may improve efficiency and as newer technology tends to improve the speed of operation. A comprehensive asset register will assist with this. It must be kept up to date, with new equipment being added and disposed equipment being removed. Occasionally, equipment may be transferred to another department. It must still be removed from one asset register and added to the register of the receiving department. A physical audit of assets usually takes place annually.

For further reading, see Assets in Action: An Asset Management Guide for Non-Technical Managers (2011), available at *www.england.nhs.uk/publication/assets-in-action-an-asset-management-guide-for-non-technical-managers.*

PROCUREMENT

Procurement is the term given to purchasing goods and services and must be supported by an appropriate business case (see Chapter 9). In a healthcare setting, these may range from small batches of catheters to large installations of equipment. There must be robust procedures in place to ensure that all purchases are 'value for money' and made within the legal framework to comply with public sector financial management and competition law.[5] In the English healthcare system, there are many guidance documents, regulations and laws associated with procurement. Although not an exhaustive list, the following documents may be useful:

- EU procurement directives and UK regulations, as many purchases may be made from European companies;[6]
- NHS England guidance on the procurement of goods;[7]
- government procurement and competition guidance;[8]
- local infection control policies, to ensure new products are compliant;
- medical devices directives, which ensure that equipment is not purchased that would negatively impact on a patient;[9]
- the Bribery Act 2010.[10]

In addition, each organisation will have its own procurement procedures comprising standardised documentation. It will also be beneficial to read the organisation's **Standing Financial Instructions** (SFIs), as these outline the financial rules, identify the management procedures and processes for purchasing goods and may include the type of business case and professional advice required to support major purchasing decisions. Recording the procurement process will provide a record of the decision for the purchase and how the purchase was made, for example through charitable funds or capital funding. Limits on the value of the purchase depend on the role of the budget holder in the organisation. It is usual that all spending is controlled through a process involving the finance department, and it will be responsible for ensuring that spending limits within an organisation's SFIs are strictly controlled. The process of assigning spending limits is often termed '**delegated authority**'. **Table 8.1** gives an example of delegated authority spending levels.

Objectives of Procurement

The purpose of the procurement process is to ensure that the most appropriate product or service is purchased. This can be summarised as follows:

- The goods are fit for the purpose for which they will be used.
- They are compliant with safety legislation and certified for use within the clinical environment, where appropriate.
- They have been purchased in the most cost-effective way to the standards stated in the specifications and the transactions have been undertaken in an open, transparent and legally compliant process.

There are many supply agreements with manufacturers for hospitals and healthcare supply of goods and services. For example, within Medical Imaging and Radiotherapy Departments these could include contrast media, catheters, thermoplastic materials, such as therapy immobilisation devices, and personal protective equipment (PPE). These purchases could be part of large-scale agreements to supply multiple products at the same price, terms and conditions to many organisations. These are termed **framework agreements**. The NHS Supply Chain (*www.supplychain.nhs.uk*) provides supplies across the service through a number of these agreements. Purchase of major capital

Table 8.1 An example of roles within the delegated authority spending limits.

Budget holder	Maximum value of authorised procurement of goods and services
Modality manager/team lead	£2,000
Service manager	£40,000
Executive director	£100,000
Director of finance	£1M
Chief executive officer	Over £1M

equipment, such as radiology or radiotherapy equipment, may be done through such a framework agreement or as an individual procurement. For consumables and smaller items, bulk purchases may be made, and the items held as stock with the supplier. This would then be ordered on a day-to-day basis as required by the clinical team.

The Stages of Procurement – Managing the Purchasing Process

High-cost items such as radiology and radiotherapy equipment will be purchased through a detailed procurement procedure for which there may be around eight stages (**Figure 8.1**). For illustration, the steps in a single procurement for a new computed tomography (CT) scanner within the NHS are outlined below.

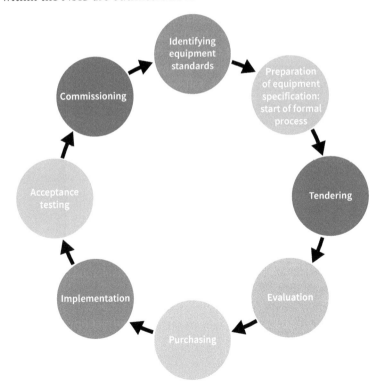

Figure 8.1 The procurement procedure.

105

1. *Identifying equipment standards.* The equipment must be purchased in line with national and international guidance and procurement law. In addition, specific technical standards applicable to radiology and radiotherapy equipment will be identified, and these must be included in the equipment specification document. This will include such technical considerations as compliance with the **Conformité Européenne** (CE) or UK Conformity Assessed (UKCA) marking requirements or other safety certifications.

2. *Preparation of equipment specification.* This is the start of the formal procurement process. The equipment specification identifies the type and technical detail of the equipment required. This may include performance standards and upgrade capability. Additionally, it may state the need for compliance with the national and international standards guidance to meet the safety standards and to operate in the clinical environment. The specification forms the basis of the **tender document**, which suppliers will use to confirm their ability to supply the equipment. For a CT scanner, this may include the following:

    - a statement of what the equipment will be used for and assessment of utilisation;
    - number of slices;
    - reconstruction parameters and algorithms;
    - gantry and size of bore;
    - table length and weight capacity;
    - power requirements;
    - room dimensions where the installation is planned;
    - a specified maximum floor loading;
    - delivery times;
    - installation project plan including pre-installation work needed;
    - warranties;
    - applications training provided by the supplier;
    - maintenance and technical support contract options;
    - phantoms and test objects provided;
    - contrast injector and respiratory gating options;
    - patient-positioning lasers.

3. *The tendering process.* The process is developed based on local rules or national frameworks of procurement and supply. This approach is to ensure openness to all companies that have the capability to supply the equipment. This openness is throughout the competitive stages, which culminate in a response to the published tender being submitted to the procurement team. This is undertaken as a series of steps from seeking interest from suppliers to the final award of a contract (**Figure 8.2**).

   a. An advertisement is issued to seek **expressions of interest** (EOIs) from suppliers. For higher-value contracts, this is done by issuing a **prior information notice** (PIN) highlighting the potential procurement or by publishing an NHS Contract Notice, formally starting the procurement and detailing how suppliers should contact the procurement team and the date for responses to be received.

   b. A **supplier questionnaire** is then issued to suppliers who have expressed an interest in bidding for the contract. This document requires the supplier to give information on the company, financial information and technical capability.

   c. On successful confirmation of the status of the company, the suppliers will be **invited to tender** (ITT) for the contract. The tender is the response by a company to supply to the specification prepared at the start of the procurement process. This will include, as a minimum, information on the equipment to be supplied, how the detailed specification stated in the tender document will be met, the price and the delivery time frame.

4. *Evaluation.* Supplier responses are assessed against the specification for meeting the requirements identified in the tender document and the price quoted. A scoring system may be used to quantify the detail of meeting the specification.

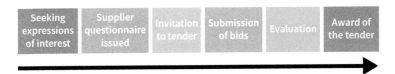

Figure 8.2 The tender process.

5. *Purchasing.* The highest-scoring bid will be purchased in line with the company's tender response. If there are several responses that meet the specification, those companies may be invited to negotiate as '**preferred bidders**' to finalise the best investment by the hospital.

6. *Implementation.* An implementation programme will be developed by the supplier. This will include such things as the delivery time and identification of any building works that will be required prior to installation. The funding for this can be substantial, especially if significant changes are being made, such as the instillation of piped anaesthetic gases, and a business case is generally required.

7. *Acceptance testing.* This is the process of confirming that the equipment is working in line with the specification and that it is operating safely. This is done with the support of technical experts, such as medical physics experts (MPEs); it will cover, for example, testing for compliance, including radiation safety (plus shielding), and safety devices, such as interlocks and emergency off switches. This is termed the '**critical examination**' and is a legal requirement under IRMER. Electrical safety will be assessed to ensure it meets the current industry regulations and infection control requirements will be identified, such as surfaces that can easily be cleaned and decontaminated.

8. *Commissioning.* The commission phase is the final stage of the installation to ensure the equipment is fully functioning. This includes the operation of the environmental systems such as heating, ventilation and emergency alarms. It may also include connection to the picture archiving and communication system (PACs), the radiology information system (RIS) and other information technology (IT) systems.

MANAGED EQUIPMENT SERVICE CONTRACTS

A managed equipment service (MES) contract is one way of procuring equipment and services; it involves contracting with one provider who has the expertise to procure, project manage, install and maintain equipment within a defined contract period, usually not less than 10 years. An **investment plan** allows for a regular cycle of replacement, enabling up-to-date equipment to be installed without multiple individual procurement bids and contracts. Financially, there is not one major outlay of money at the start of the contract as the payments are made, usually monthly, over the term of the contract. This fixed cost helps in achieving efficiency savings by reducing unwarranted variation; therefore, it enables better financial management and budget planning and negates the need to submit requests for large sums of money when equipment needs to be replaced.[5] It also enables a complete replacement plan to be generated for every piece of radiology and radiotherapy equipment within the contract. Additionally, an MES contract also provides some security within service provision as there are clear and transparent processes in the event of poor performance. Performance targets or guarantees associated with the availability of the equipment will be indicated, for example 'equipment will be functional for 98% of the time' within specified hours, usually core daytime hours. If the MES provider does not meet this target, then financial penalties apply. This results in faster response times for breakdowns for all equipment within the contract and more oversight on equipment performance as there is a requirement for regular performance reports to be issued, with improvement plans where performance has not reached the required standard. Financial penalties may also apply for poor performance outside engineer response times for faults, for example training not being delivered on time, delays in answering calls by the call centre and delays in issuing performance reports.

An MES contract can be agreed with or without the costings for associated estates work. This is the work required to prepare the room for installation, such as replacement of flooring, decoration of the walls and relocation of electrical supplies, and can be carried out by hospital contractors or as a '**turnkey project**' where the MES provider undertakes the work. Contracting without the inclusion of estates work means that a request for funding needs to be made for any work that needs to be done because of the replacements; this almost diminishes the benefits of having the contract in place. The cost of estates work when replacing equipment should not be underestimated as it can be substantial, and by including it in such contracts the risk can be significantly diminished.

Most MES providers of equipment are also manufacturers of equipment; however, the MES aspect of the company is often a subsidiary business and, as such, they offer vendor neutrality or multi-vendor provision within the contract. This means that the organisation is not tied to buying equipment only from that provider. There is a financial risk in this type of contract, but this risk lies with the MES provider. Increases in pricing of future equipment and advancements in technology, as well as the cost of ongoing maintenance, are difficult to determine for a long-term contract.

At contract negotiation, all equipment will be assigned a 'technology band' based on the needs of the service. This ranks the equipment in relation to the technology currently available, from 'high-end, state-of-the-art' equipment likely to be used for research purposes or in highly specialised departments, to the 'lower-end, day-to-day' equipment often seen as the backbone of departments. It is possible to increase the technology banding during the contract period if the service changes and requires more functionality from the equipment; however, that comes with an extra cost, which is added to the monthly payment. The banding can also be reduced. Depending on the provider, the credit released by the reduction in banding and subsequent reduction in cost of the equipment can be held by them and used to be offset against an uplift in banding on another piece of equipment or against a new piece of equipment that is to be added to the contract. Alternatively, the payments against the MES contract may be reduced. Adding or removing equipment from the contract is done through a contract variation, which is a formal process of change to the contract and agreed between the organisation and the MES provider.

The MES provider manages the procurement cycle. They will work with the organisation and medical physicists in defining the equipment specification, sourcing the appropriate equipment, disposing of old equipment, installing and commissioning the new equipment and user training. Regular investment meetings between the MES provider and the department make sure that replacements are planned in advance of the replacement date so that installations occur on time and are managed appropriately.

A typical replacement programme may look like this:

1. The person responsible for procurement in the department completes an equipment output specification as outlined above. The MES provider will check that this meets the technology banding.
2. The MES provider sends the output specification to the relevant suppliers and carries out a market evaluation of any equipment that appears to meet the requirements. It is possible to indicate which suppliers should be approached; this is beneficial if new technology has been developed by a particular supplier.
3. The market evaluation report is reviewed by the person responsible for procurement in the department and they will decide which equipment to select for user evaluation. This will involve visiting a site where the equipment is in use and assessing it against a predetermined score sheet finalised by the department and based on the output specification, but also including other elements that may have become known during the market evaluation exercise. This may be something simple, such as the weight of the equipment that needs to be handled, for example detectors or magnetic resonance coils.
4. The selected piece of equipment is approved at the investment meeting and the planning for installation commences.
5. The MES provider will oversee removal of current equipment, estates work that needs to be completed and installation of the new equipment. They will manage the commissioning, acceptance testing and applications training.

At the end of the contract period, two options are available. The organisation can purchase the equipment from the MES provider at the accounting net book value of the assets, renegotiate the contract and remain with the current provider, or transfer the equipment to a new provider.

CHAPTER SUMMARY

■ Asset management enables the status of all items of value to be seen in one place.

- There is a requirement within IRMER for an up-to-date inventory to be kept of all radiology and radiotherapy equipment.
- Procurement in healthcare is carried out within a legal framework.
- There are numerous stages of procurement, from identifying standards associated with the equipment being purchased to acceptance testing of the equipment once installed.
- Managed equipment service contracts enable an organisation to have one provider responsible for procuring and project managing equipment, with efficiency savings compared to the unwarranted variation of individual procurement projects, and performance guarantees.

REFERENCES

1. Cambridge Dictionary. Asset. Available at https://dictionary.cambridge.org/dictionary/english/asset.
2. Ionising Radiation (Medical Exposure) Regulations 2017. Available at www.legislation.gov.uk/uksi/2017/1322/contents.
3. ESR. Renewal of radiological equipment. *Insights Imaging* 2014;5:543–546.
4. COCIR. Radiotherapy Age Profile and Density. 2019. Available at www.cocir.org/fileadmin/Publications_2019/19107_COC_Radiotherapy_Age_Profile_web4.pdf.
5. HM Treasury. Managing Public Money. 2023. Available at www.gov.uk/government/publications/managing-public-money.
6. Gov.uk. EU Procurement Directives and the UK Regulations. 2017. Available at www.gov.uk/guidance/transposing-eu-procurement-directives.
7. NHS England. NHS Terms and Conditions for the Procurement of Goods and Non-clinical Service. Available at www.england.nhs.uk/nhs-terms-and-conditions-for-the-procurement-of-non-clinical-goods-and-services/.
8. Gov.uk. National Health Service (Procurement, Patient Choice and Competition) (No. 2) Regulations 2013 (Revoked). Available at www.legislation.gov.uk/uksi/2013/500/contents.
9. Gov.uk. Regulating Medical Devices in the UK. 2024. Available at www.gov.uk/guidance/regulating-medical-devices-in-the-uk.
10. Bribery Act 2010. Available at www.legislation.gov.uk/ukpga/2010/23/contents.

9. BUSINESS CASE DEVELOPMENT

Amanda Martin and Louise Kemp

INTRODUCTION

Whether it is an increase in the staffing establishment, new equipment or a major change in the infrastructure of the department, a business case is likely to be required. It may be that small projects do not require a business case and funding can be acquired through another means, such as charitable funds; however, it is unlikely that any leader or manager delivering healthcare services will not have to develop a business case during their career.

The business case is the document that provides the rationale for the request for funding and should include all of the information required by the fund holders to reach a conclusion about approving or rejecting it. It justifies the investment that is being requested and outlines the benefits in relation to the cost of the investment. A suitably constructed and written business case enables the author to consider all possible options for achieving the desired outcome.

Local business case templates may be in use, and these should be used where appropriate. However, there are generally similar key elements to all business cases, outlined in **Figure 9.1**.

DEVELOPING THE BUSINESS CASE

It is generally not possible to develop a business case in isolation. Assistance will be needed from, for example, the informatics

DOI: 9781003380078-9

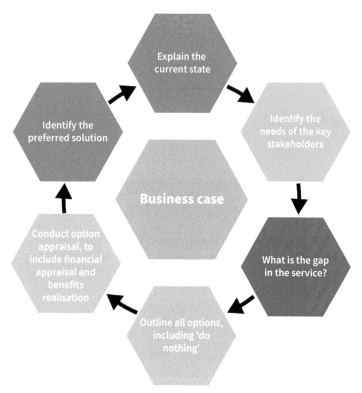

Figure 9.1 Key components of a business case.

department, the estates department and the finance team. This assistance must be sought in a timely manner, as it may take time for them to provide the information that you will need to incorporate in the business case before it is finalised.

A 'five-case model' has been developed by HM Treasury as best practice in achieving better spending decisions in public sector organisations.[1,2]

- *The strategic case*. What is the context for the proposal; why is it needed?
- *The economic case*. Does the proposal demonstrate value for money?

114

- *The commercial case.* Is the proposal viable in terms of supplier availability and procurement?
- *The financial case.* Is the proposal financially affordable?
- *The management case.* Is it possible to implement and manage the proposal?

The full five-case model approach is generally used for large-scale projects and programmes, such as new building developments, due to the high levels of investment and the scrutiny required to justify the spend. It may involve development of up to three cases, each one building upon the previous:

- *Strategic outline case* (SOC), to secure support in principle for the proposal and the case for change;
- *Outline business case* (OBC), which details the expected costs and defines the preferred option;
- *Full business case* (FBC), which is written following the procurement phase, prior to awarding a contract to the successful bidder, and confirms actual costs, timescales and implementation plans.

These cases may take many months or even years to develop, such is the level of detail and stakeholder engagement required. Most organisations will have more streamlined local business case templates for smaller projects, which will include similar information but on a more concise scale. It is important to engage with finance colleagues to ensure that the appropriate templates and submissions are used, as different templates may be required depending on the project cost.

When writing the business case, it is essential to consider the audience to which the business case will be presented; try not to use too much professional language, which may not be easily understood by those outside the medical imaging or radiotherapy department. The aim is to clearly communicate a problem that needs to be addressed, along with possible solutions, in order to secure financial support. If the reader does not understand the language, this may impact on the outcome or lead to delays in approval while details are clarified. The document must be:

- clear, without the use of jargon;
- concise, with only relevant information included;
- factual and without personal opinion.

Graphs, charts and data can be used to support the case being presented.

The format of the business case may include a number of elements; these will be summarised below.

Executive Summary

The business case starts with an executive summary, a short overview summarising the business case. It should include a brief description of the problem, the objectives of the project being proposed, the outcome required, including the benefits of the project, and the preferred option for resolving the problem. While this is often the last section to be written, it is the first section to be read by the decision-makers. It presents the whole project in an easy-to-read format without the associated detailed information found later in the business case. Smaller business cases may not require a separate executive summary as the document is already short and concise.

The Current State

This section presents the case for change: the reason why a business case is being presented and the problem that is being solved. It should describe the background to and rationale for the proposal, what the current position is and where it sits within national/regional/local/organisational contexts (e.g. alignment to relevant strategies and policies). It is important that the project being proposed is strategically aligned with the organisation's objectives and plans in its current form and with consideration of potential future changes. Data may be used to support the business case and can help the reader to visualise current and proposed states. These may be in the form of activity, equipment utilisation, staffing establishments, waiting times or demand (referral/request) data, to name just a few. It could also be data from external sources, such as the UK Model Health System, which can be used to compare local productivity to that of other similar-sized organisations.[3]

Stakeholder Consultation

A stakeholder is anyone who is affected by, or who has an interest in, the outcome of a project or service change. It is important to gain engagement from those who may be using the service currently or in the future. Stakeholder consultation is key in developing a business case that meets their needs. Chapter 11 discusses service user involvement; the benefits of involving service users in the early stages of business case development are immense. Including the experiences of service users as part of the business case narrative can be a powerful and persuasive tool. Other stakeholders must not be overlooked, for example referrers to the service, who may have significant opinions on the way the service currently works or should work in the future, or other corporate services that may be required to implement or support the service, such as housekeeping or information technology (IT) teams. Evidence of support/sign-off from stakeholders may be required as part of the case.

Gap Analysis

A gap analysis allows the gaps between the current service and the service expected by the stakeholders to be defined. It identifies the problem(s) impacting on the current service and how this will be improved or resolved by the proposed business case. Supporting documentation may include incidents that have occurred directly related to this service and risks that may be documented on the risk register, again directly related to this service.

Option Appraisal

An option appraisal is a process of reviewing possible solutions, identifying the benefits and analysing the costs so that a preferred option can be selected. Identification of the options should be carried out with all stakeholders involved. The option appraisal must include a 'do nothing' option, as this may be the preferred option once the process has been completed, or to demonstrate the cost and implications of not taking action. It is important to establish the critical criteria against which each option will be measured, including a weighting of any options that are seen to be a priority for this project. The criteria must be selected appropriately, with only those criteria that are essential for its successful delivery being included. The following may be included as critical criteria:

- **The financial impact.** This will require a financial report to be issued by the finance team, with appropriate costings for delivering the option. See below for further detail on the financial appraisal.

117

- *Value for money.* Does the option deliver improved value for money, compared with the current service?
- *Patient experience.* Will the patient experience remain the same or will it change once the option is implemented?
- *Staff experience.* Will there be any change in staff satisfaction once the option is implemented?
- *Risk.* Are there any risks associated with this option? Will any current risks be mitigated by this option?
- *Equipment utilisation.* How will this option impact on the efficiency of the equipment or service? Will there be idle time for equipment?
- *Performance.* Will activity and turnaround times be impacted if this option is selected, and to what extent?
- *Sustainability.* Will there be any future changes required in order to sustain this service?
- *Quality.* How will the quality of the service change?
- *Impact on current services.* Will this option have any impact on current services either during the implementation stages or once the project has been completed?
- *Benefits realisation.* How does this option deliver against expected benefits? See below for further detail on benefits realisation.

Financial Appraisal

The financial appraisal is usually developed with support and advice from finance partners and should define all expected costs for the proposal – how the proposal will be funded. The case should clearly articulate all costs, including peripheral and support costs over the immediate and longer term to allow a fully informed decision to be made on affordability. The following are examples of what should be included.

- *Capital requirements.* Upfront capital costs for purchasing an item of equipment or for estates/enabling works.
- *Revenue requirements.* Ongoing operational costs such as annual service charges, lease costs, subscriptions, licensing.

- **Capital charges.** Costs associated with owning an asset, such as interest charges and depreciation (an accounting charge reflecting the cost of using an asset over its predicted useful life).
- **Staff costs.** Advanced practitioner post to deliver a new service, additional portering or administrative staff needs. In business cases for additional imaging and acquisition equipment, the resource needed to report the additional cases is often overlooked.
- **Implementation costs.** Project management support, training costs.
- **Cost of each option.** Where costs of individual options differ, these should be clearly identified and easy to compare against each other. This must include the cost of doing nothing.
- **Source(s) of funding.** How does the author expect the proposal to be funded? Is funding from the organisation required? Often a business case might be expected to be supported by an existing source of finance or by a saving/efficiency delivered by the case. For example, the cost for an additional staff member may be offset by current agency or outsourcing costs, making the case cost neutral or even cost saving. Alternatively, the cost of 'do nothing' might be more expensive than the 'do something' options, particularly in the longer term.
- **Supporting information.** It may be helpful to attach quotes to support the case where appropriate.

Benefits Realisation

A benefit can be described as an outcome that adds value or leads to positive change. It is important to identify how the proposal will deliver improvements to justify the investment made, and to ensure the benefits align with the organisational strategies and objectives, particularly where public funding is used. Part of the benefits realisation is to define how benefits will be measured – how will we know if the proposal has delivered what was expected? This is an often-overlooked part of the business case and project delivery cycle, but it is important for learning lessons and providing supporting evidence for future business cases. Benefits may be tangible (measurable), such as increased activity, or intangible (not measurable), such as improved reputation. Intangible benefits can be less persuasive in terms of decision-making as they cannot be confirmed. Benefits are usually defined in terms of the following:

- *Quantitative:* cost savings, costs avoided, efficiencies, increased activity.
- *Qualitative:* improved patient or staff experience, higher-quality images – more accurate diagnoses.

Benefits can be more compelling if they are specific; for example, in making a case for a new X-ray room: 'expansion in appointment numbers' is difficult to quantify, but 'an additional 20 appointments/day, increasing capacity by 25% and reducing current outpatient X-ray waiting times from 9 days to 5 days' gives a much clearer indication of the impact.

It may be helpful to include evidence of the expected benefits, such as real-world data or precedents set by similar projects, to support the credibility of the claims.

Identify the Preferred Option

Once the option appraisal has been completed and scored, one or more options are likely to be identified as having the potential to deliver the objectives outlined earlier. A strengths, weaknesses, opportunities and threats (SWOT) analysis can be carried out to support the decision for the preferred option. An option that scores highly may be excluded due to external constraints such as legal or regulatory requirements that cannot be overcome, making it an unviable option. **Table 9.1** presents an example of how to develop a business case for the purchase of a new mobile fluoroscopy unit.

The Approvals Process

The finished business case will need to be submitted to the appropriate forum with the ability to approve the proposal and associated financial arrangements. It is the job of the approving body to determine whether the proposal delivers sufficient benefits, is aligned to objectives, is deliverable, is affordable and is value for money against the resources available.

The business case approval process may be defined in the organisation's Standing Financial Instructions (SFIs) and/or the business case

Table 9.1 An example of a business case development for the purchase of a new mobile fluoroscopy machine.

Business case stage	Example
The current state	What is the purpose of the mobile fluoroscopy unit in this context? Why is a new one required? Is it a replacement, a response to increased demand or to develop a new service/procedure?
Stakeholder consultation	Patients, Radiology and Orthopaedics Departments, theatre and other medical specialties involved in the proposed service, support services such as radiation protection advisor, IT team, estates.
Gap analysis	Details of what can be done presently versus what could be done with the new machine, for example currently insufficient trauma theatre capacity to meet demand, meaning longer waiting times for trauma cases; affects 'X' number of patients/week.
Option appraisal	These may include outsourcing to another provider, purchasing up front and leasing. It must include the do-nothing option.
Financial appraisal	Include such cost(s) as the financial cost of the new machine, installation costs, annual service charges, increased staffing requirements of, for example, additional radiographer hours, IT connectivity, licence or support staff costs, new data point or power supplies in theatre, additional lead aprons, additional support from the medical physics experts.
Benefits realisation	These may be reduced number of breakdowns (fewer service interruptions), reduced staff/patient dose, delivery of a new service and associated improvement in delivery of diagnostics or treatments, additional theatre capacity of 'X' cases per week, reduced waiting lists.
Identify the preferred option	Select an option that is commercially and financially viable and that will meet the expectations of the future service. Include reasons for this being the preferred option.

policy. The group that, or individual who, can approve a business case will usually vary depending on the cost of the proposal. For example, a business case for a £20,000 workstation might be approved at divisional board level, a £300,000 IT system could require approval from the director of finance and a £900,000 magnetic resonance (MR) scanner might need to be signed off by the health board. Very high-value (multimillion pound) cases may also need sign-off at regional health board or government level, such as a radiotherapy satellite suite. Additionally, a business case may have to pass through a number of different boards or levels of approval to reach final sign-off. This is to ensure that appropriate scrutiny has been applied at specialty/divisional level, so that cases that reach the finance director and executive team are fit for purpose. The input of a 'critical reader' or internal expert panel may be beneficial in refining the business case document by providing valuable feedback on content and format before submitting for approval. It is good practice to 'socialise' business cases prior to submission for approval, particularly in higher-value cases. This ensures that the approving group/individual expecting to review the case can flag any concerns or queries and has a reasonable understanding of the proposal and expected cost in advance, which can help smooth the path to approval.

CHAPTER SUMMARY

- The business case is a document that supports a request for funding.
- It should include all relevant information required by the decision-makers in order for them to reach a decision.
- It justifies the investment that is being requested.
- It should address the strategic, economic, commercial, financial and management cases.
- It should be written in a clear and concise format.
- The executive summary is a short overview of the business case.

FURTHER READING

- The Healthcare Financial Management Association (HFMA) offers short courses in the development of business cases: www.hfma.org.uk/education-items/nhs-business-cases-england.
- NHS Property Services. Your Guide to Building a Business Case. Available at www.property.nhs.uk/news/blogs/your-guide-to-building-a-business-case/.

REFERENCES

1. HM Treasury. The Green Book: Appraisal and Evaluation in Central Government. 2022. Available at www.gov.uk/government/publications/the-green-book-appraisal-and-evaluation-in-central-government.
2. Welsh Government. Guide to Developing the Project Business Case. 2018. Available at www.gov.wales/sites/default/files/publications/2018-08/guide-to-developing-the-project-business-case.pdf.
3. NHS England. The Model Health System. Available at www.england.nhs.uk/applications/model-hospital/.

SECTION 3
SERVICE DEVELOPMENT

10. CONTINUOUS QUALITY IMPROVEMENT

Lesley Wright

INTRODUCTION

Radiographers, through their training, are skilled to produce an excellent radiographic image or provide therapy treatment. However, the current training schemes do not provide radiographers with the skills to understand how to get the best from the resources and meet the requirements of the service, whether it is the whole service or a single modality. To deliver highly effective and efficient services, it is important to understand the factors that influence the flow of patients through the patient pathway (patient flow). For Medical Imaging and Radiotherapy Departments, this commences when the referral is received (**Figure 10.1**); however, it must be recognised that this may be some way along the patient pathway. Events occurring prior to the referral may influence a patient's diagnostic or therapy experience. Equally important is having the knowledge and tools, including those associated with capacity, demand and flow, to be able to continuously improve as the requirements of the services change.

This chapter will start with a list of helpful definitions, which you can refer to as you progress through the chapter.

DOI: 9781003380078-10

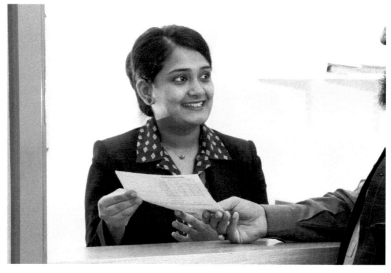

Figure 10.1 Receipt of a medical imaging referral.

DEFINITIONS

Activity is the number of patients/examinations completed in a defined period of time; the unit of measure is patients or examinations per unit of time.

Backlog/work in progress (WIP) is the number of examinations or patients, often referred to as a queue or inventory. Backlog or WIP is a very useful process metric to use for monitoring because it reacts quickly to changes and is relatively sensitive to demand and activity variation, and so provides a good early warning signal.

Batching is a policy constraint that schedules all tasks to arrive at the same time, or allows tasks to be stored and released at the same time. This creates bottlenecks and results in poor flow.

Capacity is a generic term. There are many types of capacity, including skill capacity and slot capacity. Skill capacity is those skills required for flow, for example insertion of Venflon™ or reporting. Slot capacity is the number of slots required to meet the demand. Each form of capacity has a different unit of measure. In medical imaging and radiotherapy, we usually measure 'resource-time capacity' in hours.

Carve-out is when available capacity is ring-fenced, reserved for specific examinations, priorities, referral sources or even consultants. Each slot is then operated independently. If there is any variation in demand or load, then the effect of carve-out is to increase the total capacity required to achieve the same service quality. Carve-out can apply to any form of capacity, including space, resource time, slot and flow, and multiple forms of carve-out can coexist and aggravate each other.

Circle of control is those staff who are involved in a process that they have the power to change and influence.

Circle of influence is those staff who are not directly involved in a process, but have the power to influence, for example senior leaders or head of portering services.

Circle of concern is those staff or organisations not directly involved in a process, but which are responsible for monitoring, for example an organisation's management board, the Care Quality Commission (CQC) or a professional body.

Cycle time is the time interval between starting one patient and being ready to start the next patient. The unit of measurement is time, in minutes. When measuring the cycle time, it is useful to view patient flow through the room on a Gantt chart. Cycle times can be used to establish the appointment interval slots. Adding the total cycle times together over a period of time, such as 1 day, will give the total load on the system.

Demand is the number of patients/examinations that arrive in a defined period of time: the unit of measure is patients or examinations per unit of time.

Effectiveness is the degree to which the service achieves its intended outcome. Effectiveness can be quantified only if the intended outcome is defined, and the actual outcome is measured. Effectiveness is calculated from the ratio of the count of successes to the count of attempts, as a percentage.

Efficiency is a measure of the degree to which the service does not waste resources; 100% efficiency implies zero waste. Efficiency is measured independently of effectiveness, though both are the effects of the same system design, measured as a percentage.

Flow capacity is the number of tasks that can be processed in a defined interval of time.

Hand-off is the transfer of a task from one step or person to another.

Lead time is the interval between two events, for example date and time of request to date and time of scan, or date and time of scan to date and time of report. End-to-end lead time is date and time of request to date and time of report.

Policy constraint is something that limits the form or function of a system. Policy constraints are often assumptions and beliefs that are introduced to improve the process, but frequently have a detrimental impact. The most common policy constraints are time traps, batching and carve-out (TTBACO) (see definitions).

Productivity is a single measure of the performance of a process or system; it combines both effectiveness and efficiency, that is, productivity = effectiveness × efficiency. Productivity can be improved by improving effectiveness (increasing quality) or by improving efficiency (reducing waste). Productivity is a dimensionless ratio with a range of 0–100%.

Patient flow is the rate of movement through a process or system.

Resource-time capacity is used to measure the capacity of a room, and the ability to undertake an examination/treatment; it includes staff and equipment. A scanner without staff is not capacity.

Segmentation is the separation of the whole process of care for one group of patients, but not at the expense of other patients.

Time trap is a process design (policy constraint) that ensures that the lead time is independent of the flow, for example booking all routine patients who should be imaged within 6 weeks at 42 days, ignoring empty booking slots. It pushes the patient to the furthest point, rather than pulling them forward. A time trap can also be caused by carve-out of urgent or 2-week wait (2WW) slots.

Touch time is the time that a resource/staff 'touches' the patient/task. It is a component of cycle time, but does not include the change-over time, which would include cleaning a room or changing a coil, for example.

Utilisation is the ratio of the time that a resource (scanner and staff) is busy (i.e. not idle), divided by the time that the resource (scanner and staff) is available; it is expressed as a percentage. High efficiency implies high utilisation, but high utilisation does not imply high efficiency, as utilisation can include waste.

Validate is the act of testing to demonstrate fitness for purpose, that is, does the data, product or service meet the needs of the customer in full, on time and at an affordable cost, and provide the value intended to the stakeholders?

Value is the worth of a product or service as perceived by the customer and enjoyed by the stakeholders of the system when the system is in operation.

Verification is the act of testing that a product or service has been built according to the design specification and requirements.

WHAT IS CONTINUOUS QUALITY IMPROVEMENT?

Continuous quality improvement (CQI) is used by organisations to make changes by continuously adapting and refining processes. CQI can be known by other terms and use different methodologies. Of the many terms used, the following are the more familiar ones:

- healthcare systems engineering (HCSE);
- Lean/Six Sigma;
- quality, service improvement and redesign (QSIR);
- theory of constraints.

The principle of any improvement effort should:

- put the patient at the heart of everything we do;
- be clinically led, with management support;
- be supported by validated data;
- ensure that technical improvement expertise is designed to build in-house capability and lifelong learning;
- ensure that sustainability is built into the Medical Imaging and Radiotherapy Departments, and the way in which these departments work.

As a leader or manager of a service or modality, it is important to understand how to get the best from the resources you manage. Resources within a healthcare environment may include the following:

- staff;
- medical imaging or radiotherapy equipment;
- supplies such as catheters, cannulas and materials for making therapy moulds;
- contrast agents and other drugs;
- patient monitoring equipment;
- waiting areas, administrative areas and clinical rooms.

Critical to this is understanding patient flow. A patient's pathway will have started before they arrive in the Medical Imaging and Radiotherapy Departments, via general practice, the Emergency Department (ED), an inpatient (IP) ward, the Outpatient Department (OPD) or another healthcare provider. Only the patient and their carer will understand the whole patient journey, including any delays and frustrations.

FOCUS FOR IMPROVEMENT

Any improvement effort needs to align with the strategic aims of the organisation, which, in turn, are aligned with the NHS priorities and strategies, often laid out in new publications.

- In 2019, NHS England (NHSE) published Transforming Imaging Services in England: A National Strategy for Imaging.[1] Imaging networks are now well established across England.
- In 2020, Diagnostics: Recovery and Renewal[2] significantly shaped the direction for all diagnostics by recommending five key priority areas, including the establishment of Community Diagnostic Centres (CDCs).
- From 2020, Radiology: Getting It Right First Time (GIRFT)[3] makes 20 recommendations to help maximise existing capacity and plan for expansion, with the creation of CDCs away from hospital sites.
- The annual Priorities and Operational Planning Guidance[4] sets out the key annual priorities and objectives for each part of the NHS.

It is important to be clear on the focus of improvement, for example the problem to solve (e.g. following a complaint) or the key target to be met (e.g. monthly diagnostic waiting times and activity for 15 diagnostic tests, commonly called DM01[5,6]).

The improvement could focus on any of the following:

- **Patients:**
  - improving waiting times for examinations and results;
  - minimising waits and delays;
  - offering choice of appointments;
  - providing an extended-hours service;
  - reducing multiple visits;

- **Staff:**
  - removing duplication, such as appointment cancellations;
  - planning services more effectively;
  - increasing skills;
  - reducing interruptions, calm environment;

- **Organisation:**
  - improving productivity;
  - saving money from outsourcing, overtime, waiting list initiatives (WLIs);
  - achieving NHS targets and key performance indicators (KPIs);
  - reducing complaints;
  - using underutilised capacity, increasing activity to reduce cost per test;
  - service expansion.

IMPROVEMENT METHODOLOGIES

There are several improvement methodologies, but most are based on the following:

- **Lean.** Lean[7] is a term that was introduced when a study was conducted on the Toyota philosophy of the management and culture it had created among workers to improve processes. It is widely used in manufacturing. It focuses on the continuous elimination of waste: transport, inventory, motion, waiting, overproduction, overprocessing, defects and skills (TIMWOODS). It has five key steps.

1. Specify **value** from the customer's point of view.
2. Identify the **value stream** and identify waste.
3. Make value **flow**.
4. Supply what is **pulled** by the customer.
5. Continually improve and strive for **perfection**.

- ◼ ***Six Sigma.*** Six Sigma was developed in manufacturing. It is a rigorous strategy for improvement based on analysis and measurement. Six Sigma aims to develop products and services to such a high level of reliability that they are virtually 'defect free'. The methodology is called DMAIC: define, measure, analyse, improve and control. It is not widely used in healthcare.
- ◼ ***Healthcare systems engineering.***[8] Systems engineering is an interdisciplinary field of engineering and engineering management that focuses on how to design, integrate and manage complex systems. Used in aerospace, it is now being applied in healthcare, which also has complex systems. It provides a framework and methodology for improving safety, flow, quality and productivity (SFQP). It is evidence based and data driven.
- ◼ ***Theory of constraints.*** The theory of constraints is a management philosophy that helps identify the crucial limiting factor (usually referred to as a constraint or a bottleneck) that stands in the way of achieving a goal. The main goal of the theory of constraints is to lessen the constraint to the point where it is no longer the limiting factor.

DEVELOPING IMPROVEMENT STRATEGIES

Before starting any improvement effort, it is important to ask the following questions.

- ◼ What is the problem to be solved?
- ◼ What is the diagnosis?
- ◼ Where is the evidence to support the diagnosis?

- How will we know that a change is an improvement? Any improvement is a change, but not every change is an improvement.
- How does the improvement align with the key goals and visions for the department and the organisation?

Developing a Team Approach to Improvement

Improvement efforts require change, and change is a challenge for most people, with many fearful of it. Implementing and sustaining change is more likely if those impacted by the change help to shape what the change will be, rather than have it imposed upon them. Before starting, and depending on the focus for improvement, bring together a multidisciplinary team that reflects all involved in the process (**circle of control**; see Figure 10.7), for example booking clerks, radiographers, healthcare assistants, radiologists and nurses. Each will have a different view of the patient pathway and no one person will completely understand what it entails. The problem to solve may arise in a different part of a wider patient pathway. It will be important to identify additional staff who might be in the **circle of influence** (see Figure 10.7), as you may need to involve them in the improvement process early on.

Leadership

The role of a leader is to set direction, open up possibilities, help people achieve, communicate and deliver. It is also about behaviour – what leaders do is more important than what they say. The challenge for leading improvement is in developing a culture of continuous improvement, as identified by NHS Improving Patient Care Together (NHS IMPACT).[9] It should be a core activity for senior leaders and clinicians, with time built in for staff to learn the methodologies and to take part in **tests of change**, which should happen before implementing significant changes. The impact can be assessed to see if a positive difference has been made. Agreeing a set of measures before and after the change will help in understanding the impact objectively rather than subjectively. Some changes may take time to have an impact, for example making changes in a booking system may take time to show any improvement due to patients already booked. Review the measures of

135

any changes regularly then come together to reflect on the impact and use the data to plan the next test of change.

Executive Support

Medical Imaging and Radiotherapy Departments will benefit from having executive support, such as a senior leader, possibly a director with responsibility for CQI, whose role will be to ensure that the improvement is aligned with the strategic vision and to remove barriers by influencing senior staff to support the change. Some organisations will have an improvement department; however, it is important that leaders have the skills to make their own improvements and be in control of the services they deliver.

Managing Change

Remember that any improvement is a change, but not every change is necessarily an improvement. A change can be perceived as a threat to security, and this will give rise to emotional resistance. Ensure that the voices of those who may not see the need for change are heard, but these should be counterbalanced with evidence and data, and with encouragement for ideas from all staff. **Figure 10.2** shows the 'nerve

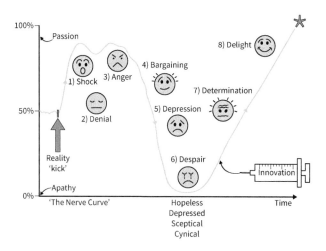

Figure 10.2 Nerve curve. (Courtesy of Simon Dodds.)

curve', which demonstrates the emotional journey involved in making successful change; it is based on the work of E. Kübler-Ross.[10]

UNDERSTANDING PATIENT FLOW

Many problems associated with poor flow are caused by poor processes, unnecessary steps that add no value and the impact of **policy constraints** (human-made rules), such as TTBACO. All these increase variation in lead times and impact patient flow. To manage your service effectively, you need to have access to the following:

- weekly demand;
- weekly activity;
- backlog;
- lead times (request to scan, scan to report);
- cancellation and 'did not attend' (DNA) rates.

It is important to understand the relationship between these metrics. Are the above data readily available? Do you have access to them on a weekly basis? Are they visible to all staff, not hidden away on a computer? Have the data been validated? Validation is a quality process that seeks to determine if the data are fit for purpose, and contain all the patients, dates and referral sources, for example. The radiology information system (RIS) lead or business intelligence (BI) lead will play a key part in providing these data. Establishing a clinical dashboard is a great place to start. A clinical dashboard should provide a visual display of the key data required to manage the service, an example of which can be seen in Figure 10.4, and ideally be refreshed weekly. The dashboard should be placed somewhere in the department where staff can easily view it. A simple notice board would be ideal, rather than only on a computer where it might be out of sight. It can also contain information on current improvements being tested.

Basics of Flow Science – Demand and Capacity

The analogy of flow through a bath (**Figure 10.3**) will be used to explain patient flow through the computed tomography (CT) service from receipt of request to scan.

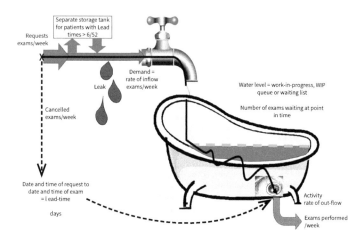

Figure 10.3 Diagram of flow through CT 'bath'. (Courtesy of Dr Kate Silvester.)

The requests arrive in the CT Department, are vetted and sorted into two groups:

1. Patients who need a CT scan within 6 weeks and are subject to the DM01, cancer targets, ED and IP delivery targets.
2. Patients who do not need a CT scan within 6 weeks and are not subject to the DM01 target. These are follow-up or surveillance requests for patients with known pathology and are 'diverted' and held into a separate 'planned tank' within the RIS so that their longer lead times do not 'contaminate' the DM01 performance data. Patients due their CT scans in the following month are then 'released' from this separate tank and join the stream of DM01 patients to be booked. At this point, there is a 'leak' (indicated in red in Figure 10.3) when appointments are cancelled by the patient or hospital. All the patients leaking from the system need to be 'gathered up' and rebooked. This involves disruptive rework for the booking and vetting staff, with delays and clinical risk for these patients.

Other patients, that is, those not subject to DM01 or to a 'planned' examination, flow through the 'tap' (demand) to be held in 'the bath' (booked waiting list) ready to go through the scanner 'plug hole' (activity). The flow through the 'tap' and 'plug hole' is controlled by the department's operational policies, such as time traps, batching and carve-out.

- If the average demand (flow through the tap) equals the average activity (flow though the plug hole), then the waiting list/WIP (level of the bath water) will stay constant.
- If the demand is greater than the activity, the waiting list (level of the bath water) will increase.
- If the activity is greater than the demand, the waiting list (level of the bath water) will reduce.

Figure 10.4 is a CT Diagnostic Vitals Chart® (DVC); this shows the relationship between the weekly requests or demand, including cancellations (blue); weekly images or activity (orange); weekly work in progress (WIP) (broken green); and weekly cancellations (red). The WIP line is the most sensitive to change. The chart shows the WIP is reducing slowly over time. Once the cancellations have been subtracted

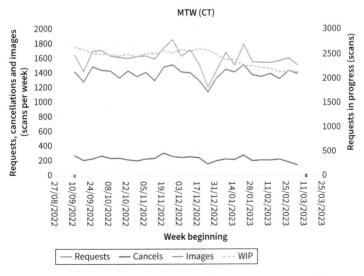

Figure 10.4 CT Diagnostic Vitals Chart®: weekly requests, images, WIP and cancellations. (Courtesy Maidstone and Tunbridge Wells NHS Trust.)

from the requests (demand), the reduction in the WIP is due to the activity being greater than the demand. The requests (demand) and activity both show some natural variation, with the expected reduction over a bank holiday. The y-axis on the right (WIP) is a higher scale (0–3000) than the y-axis on the left (requests, cancellations and images per week) (0–2000). Observing a simple set of weekly data will quickly alert the senior leader to any changes that could have an impact on service delivery.

BASIC TOOLS AND TECHNIQUES FOR DELIVERING IMPROVEMENT

Walk the Pathway

Before learning the variety of different tools available to support the methodology you are using, one of the most critical and valuable steps is to 'walk the walk' of the patient and their carer. Walk the pathway from the moment the patient is referred; this may be within the hospital or from primary care. Put yourself in the shoes of the patient and their carer so that you can understand their experience. Start from the beginning and ask yourself how easy it is to park or find the Medical Imaging or Radiotherapy Department, for example. Your improvement effort may be the result of a complaint, with the complainant seeing things differently to those who are delivering the service. Each staff member will understand the process from their perspective; however, the patient and carer will experience and feel the impact of each process. Improvement cannot be done from an office.

Mapping

There are several maps that can be produced; each has a different purpose and will add value to the improvement effort.

System Map

Figure 10.5 is a high-level system map depicting the flow of patients from referral to reporting. This is typical of many organisations with

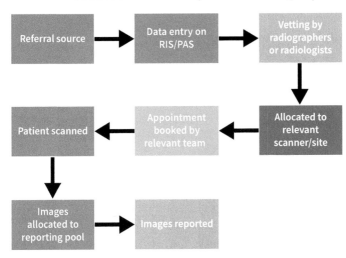

Figure 10.5 System map demonstrating referral to imaging.

more than one site. Elective referrals come from general practice, the OPD, the ED, IP clinicians and, occasionally, from outside the organisation. The patient data and requests are input into the RIS and a patient management system or patient administration system (PAS) if they have not previously attended the organisation. They are vetted to ensure that the request is justified; next, a scanner and site are selected and an appointment is generated. The patient is then imaged, and the images reported.

Process Map

Figure 10.6 is an example of a process map. It is in greater detail than the system map. It visualises a series of connected steps and covers the agreed start and end points of the improvement effort (scope).

The process map highlights the number, and types, of steps in the process:

- value-added steps from the patient's perspective (green squares);
- steps performed to facilitate the scan (blue squares);
- unnecessary waits between process steps (red stars);
- the one necessary wait for the blood test result (purple star).

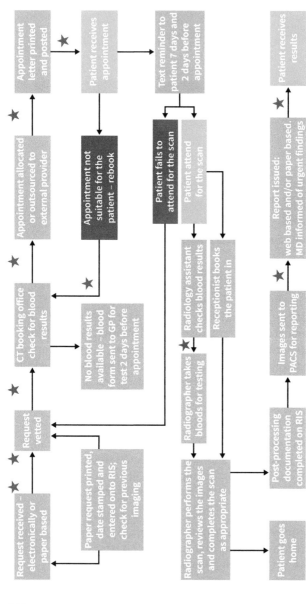

Figure 10.6 Process map demonstrating receipt of referral to the referrer receiving the report. GP, general practitioner; MDT, multidisciplinary team; PACS, picture archiving and communication system.

When creating the process map, it is essential to include all those involved in the process. Rarely does any one single person understand every single step. What is thought to happen is often very different in reality, and many steps and processes evolve over time. There are many opportunities for delays and errors as information and tasks are passed between staff.

Stakeholder Map

There will be many people (stakeholders) who have an interest in the outcomes of the improvement effort, all for very different reasons. A stakeholder map (**Figure 10.7**) adds value by demonstrating the relationship each of these has to each other. Central to all improvement efforts are the patient and carer, and there are three stakeholder groups who surround them.

Those in the 'circle of control' should have a deep understanding of the process required to get the desired result. Those in the 'circle of influence' should have some understanding of the process and will often influence the policies, such as waiting-list policies. Those in the 'circle of concern' are concerned about the performance and control at a strategic or national level. By documenting and understanding these relationships, when you want to make a 'test of change' that is outside the 'circle of control', the stakeholder map will provide an understanding of who to approach for help and who can influence change.

Measurement

Why measure? How do we know if we have made an improvement? Only by undertaking a baseline measurement before the improvement effort starts and measuring again after a 'test of change' can you understand the impact of change, but keep measures specific, measurable, achievable, relevant and time-bound (SMART). The measures will depend on the scope of the project; for example, if you are looking to improve patient flow from request to imaging or treatment, then the measure will be 'time', from the date and time of the request until the date and time of the imaging or treatment.

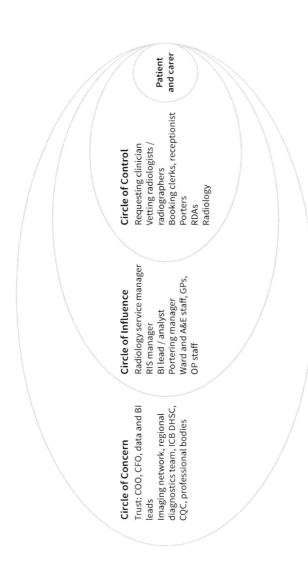

Circle of Concern

Trust: COO, CFO, data and BI leads
Imaging network, regional diagnostics team, ICB DHSC, CQC, professional bodies

Circle of Influence

Radiology service manager
RIS manager
BI lead / analyst
Portering manager
Ward and A&E staff, GPs, OP staff

Circle of Control

Requesting clinician
Vetting radiologists / radiographers
Booking clerks, receptionist
Porters
RDAs
Radiology

Patient and carer

Figure 10.7 Stakeholder map. A&E, Accident and Emergency; CFO, chief financial officer; COO, chief operating officer; DHSC, Department of Health and Social Care; GP, general practitioner; ICB, integrated care board; OP, outpatient; RDA, Radiology Department assistant.

Variation

Variation occurs in most processes; however, we can make the variation worse by the way we organise processes, for example batching requests, vetting, appointments and reporting. Artificial variation has much more of an impact on patient flow than natural variation. Common-cause variation is normal and expected. Special-cause variation produces unusual or unexpected variations in a system. If you measure the time it takes to get from home to work, it will vary slightly every day. If you have a punctured tyre, it will take much longer to get to work, but this happens only rarely; this is an example of a special-cause variation.

The key to improving patient flow is reducing variation. An effective way to measure variation is to use a **statistical process control (SPC) chart**. This is a simple graphic tool that enables a process to be measured (**Figures 10.8** and **10.9**). **Figure 10.8** shows the variation in lead times for magnetic resonance imaging (MRI) for consecutive patients from receipt of request to scan for patients on a cancer 2WW pathway. The y-axis is days (0–80), and the x-axis is consecutive patients over a 3-month period. The green horizontal line demonstrates a mean of 24 days, the blue line is the 14-day target and the red line is the upper control limit (UCL), which is 3 standard deviations from the mean. There is significant variation in lead times and most patients are not imaged within 14 days.

If the focus for improvement is to improve reporting times for routine outpatients, an SPC chart can be used as a baseline. **Figure 10.9** shows the variation in CT reporting lead times (image to report) for consecutive routine patients over time. The y-axis is days (0–30 days), and the x-axis is consecutive patients over a 1-month period. The variation is 0–27 days, with a mean of 4.7 days. The red line is the UCL, which is 3 standard deviations from the mean.

When we have significant variation in lead times, it makes planning the next step in the patient pathway very difficult. An effective pathway requires guaranteed and predictable lead times. Failure to provide this could mean wasted outpatient appointments, with results not available at the point of consultation.

Keep measures high level and simple; a few good-quality measures are better than a plethora of poorly collated ones.

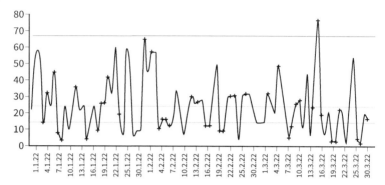

Figure 10.8 Variation in MRI lead times from receipt of request to scan for consecutive patients on the 2 week wait pathway.

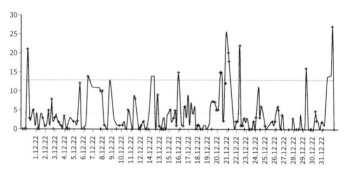

Figure 10.9 Variation in CT lead times from consecutive patients from completion of scan to report being issued.

Cycle Times

Measuring cycle times provides evidence of how long a specific process takes, from the start of one cycle of the process to being ready to start the next cycle. Cycle times can be used to measure the utilisation of a resource, such as a CT scanner, and therefore allows the correct scheduling of patient appointment slots. The cycle time is measured from the time a patient walks into the room until the room/staff are ready to receive the next patient. Each patient will have a different cycle time. Cycle times are measured by examination type; the mean cycle time for a particular examination type should be calculated, allowing a correct appointment time slot allocation to be made. Cycle times can reduce if the process changes; for example, updated software can shorten the acquisition time, or cannulation undertaken outside the room will reduce the cycle time. Collecting cycle time data at the point of source will provide an insight into the time it takes for the whole process; it must include the essential time required to clean the room or to change an MRI coil. Capture the cycle times over an operational week, for example 8.00–20.00, 7 days a week, as this will give a good insight into patient flow. From these data, it is then possible to visualise the patient flow using a **Gantt chart**. A Gannt chart is a bar chart that demonstrates where work has been completed over a period of time. The Gantt chart in **Figure 10.10** represents what is happening in a CT scanning room:

- *green bar* – patient is in the scanning room;
- *yellow bar* – the scanner is being cleaned;
- *orange bar* – no patient activity in the scanning room.

This shows the patient flow, demonstrating a late start at the beginning of the day (red), and differences between the appointment time allocation and the examination cycle time.

Cycle times can also be used to determine how much staff time is required to undertake a certain role. For example, if you are planning to expand a reception to book in patients, measure the cycle times of booking patients over the period of a day; this will provide the mean time it takes to book a patient. You can then calculate how many patients can be booked in each hour. It is important to remember that no resource can be busy 100% of the time.

Workload

The workload on an imaging room or radiotherapy room can be measured by adding together all the individual patient cycle times for the day.

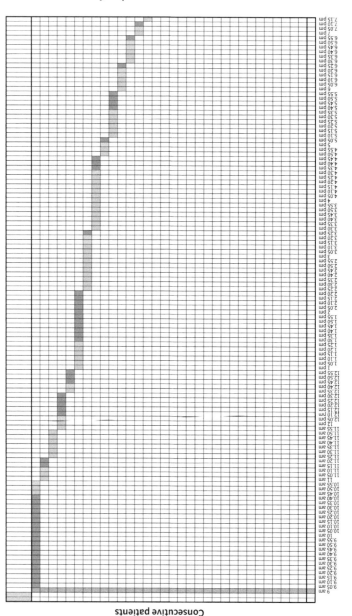

Figure 10.10 Daily Gantt chart for CT.

Consecutive patients

Utilisation

Using the load and operating-hours data, the percentage utilisation of a scanner/room can be measured (**Table 10.1**). Utilisation is the time the resource (staffed scanner) is busy, including prep and cleaning, divided by the time it is available, expressed as a percentage. Complex imaging or treatments will have long cycle times; therefore, the number of patients imaged is not a good measure of utilisation. It is possible to have a small number of patients with a high utilisation, or a large number of patients and low utilisation. Utilisation is not necessarily a measure of effectiveness, as a resource can be busy performing non-value-added work, such as cannulating a patient on the CT table rather than outside the room.

In summary, to calculate utilisation, the following are required:

- *Cycle times*: for every patient for each day for a period (e.g. 7 days);
- *Load*: sum of the cycle times in hours and minutes each day;
- *Operating hours*: staffed scanner (resource capacity) time in hours and minutes per day for the same period of time;
- *Activity*: number of patients imaged each day for the same period of time.

Table 10.1 Activity, load, operational hours and utilisation.

Scanner	8 June 2021	9 June 2021	10 June 2021	11 June 2021	12 June 2021
Number of patients	36	35	38	34	42
Load	7 hours 10 minutes	7 hours 17 minutes	8 hours 38 minutes	8 hours 53 minutes	8 hours 34 minutes
Operating hours	12 hours	12 hours	12 hours	12 hours	12 hours
% Utilisation	59.72%	60.69%	71.94%	74.03%	71.39%

UNDERSTANDING POLICY CONSTRAINTS

Policy constraints are assumptions and beliefs that have been introduced to try and improve the process, but unwittingly can make the lead times longer and will create variation. When looking at any process, it is likely that policy constraints will have been introduced. The main policy constraints are TTBACO.

Time Traps

An example of a time trap is when a routine patient with a request to be completed within 6 weeks is booked at 42 days, even though there are other empty slots available. This is shown in **Figure 10.11**, where each black dot is the time a patient was imaged from the request being made; the dense cluster of black dots demonstrates where patients have been booked at 6 weeks, whereas the lack of black dots below demonstrates earlier slots that were not used.

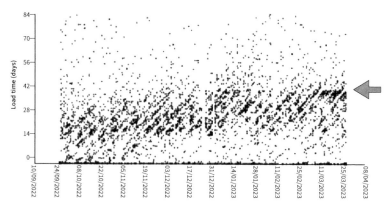

Figure 10.11 Lead times (request to scan) showing a 42-day time trap.

Batching

Batching is a human-made policy constraint that occurs when tasks or patients are grouped and processed together; for example, in Medical Imaging and Radiotherapy Departments, batching may occur in vetting, scheduling, reporting and downloading data. External to Medical Imaging and Radiotherapy Departments, it could be batching of referrals at the end of a ward round or clinic. Batching is felt to be more efficient, waiting until there are enough tasks waiting rather than doing one single task as soon as it arrives. However, the opposite applies: batching creates bottlenecks and causes poor flow and delays. From a patient's perspective, batching results in the first patient or task in the queue waiting for enough patients or tasks to arrive before the first patient/task is acted on. For example, batching of vetting, perhaps until the end of the day, can result in the booking staff waiting to process appointments; the appointments are then delayed or slots are unable to be filled, impacting lead times and patient flow. The ideal process is little and often; as a result, the impact of delays cannot be felt.

Carve-out

This is a very common policy constraint whereby a patient is given priority, or a slot is ring-fenced for a certain group of patients or for specific conditions. The impact will be to push one group of patients through the system faster, resulting in other patients waiting longer. This can significantly increase waiting times; then, as waiting times grow, referrers increase the number of patients they request as 'urgent' or 'high priority'. The process then becomes a vicious circle that is difficult to manage. Carve-out will result in additional capacity being required to deliver the service. The following are examples of carve-out:

- Appointment slots carved out for 2WWs, one-stop clinics, urgent scans or scans that specific consultants want allocated to a specific 'session'.
- Staff reporting examinations may choose to report certain types of examinations before others, prioritising patient groups; for example, an outpatient before a general practice referral. They may also prioritise certain reports due to personal preference, such as reporting easier, short examinations rather than longer, complex

examinations, or choosing to prioritise certain body parts due to having a specific interest. In addition, the reporter may report images only when they are allocated to their work sessions.

It is often necessary to prioritise some reports, such as IP or ED before outpatient reports, or if staff have specific skills or knowledge for complex imaging procedures. In each case, patients should be taken in order where appropriate. **Figure 10.12** shows an example of a CT scheduling week; each colour represents when specific scans can be booked. If the specific appointment slot occurs only once a week, the patient may have to wait longer for an appointment. The impact of carve-out is to create significant variation in the lead time from request to examination, examination to report, and the end to end lead times from patient request to report. This makes it difficult for a referring clinician to book the next step in the pathway, such as the next outpatient or general practitioner (GP) appointment, due to lack of guaranteed and predictable turnaround times. Variation in the end-to-end lead times could result in the patient attending an outpatient clinic and no result is available. The clinic and patients are then delayed while the clinic calls the department to get an urgent report, or the patient leaves the clinic and is required to return later. Lead times for imaging and reporting should be monitored on a regular basis and shared with colleagues via a clinical dashboard, as previously discussed (Figures 10.8 and 10.9). Staff could be unaware that they are causing unwarranted variation unless the data are monitored and discussed.

Segmentation

There are occasions when it is necessary to see some patients at a specific time, but not at the expense of other patients. This might include patients requiring a general anaesthetic, whereby certain equipment or expert staff are available only at a certain time. The slots allocated need to be in proportion to the demand to ensure that those patients are not advantaged or disadvantaged by being seen sooner or waiting longer than other patients. When introducing segmentation, it is necessary to look at the whole scheduling system.

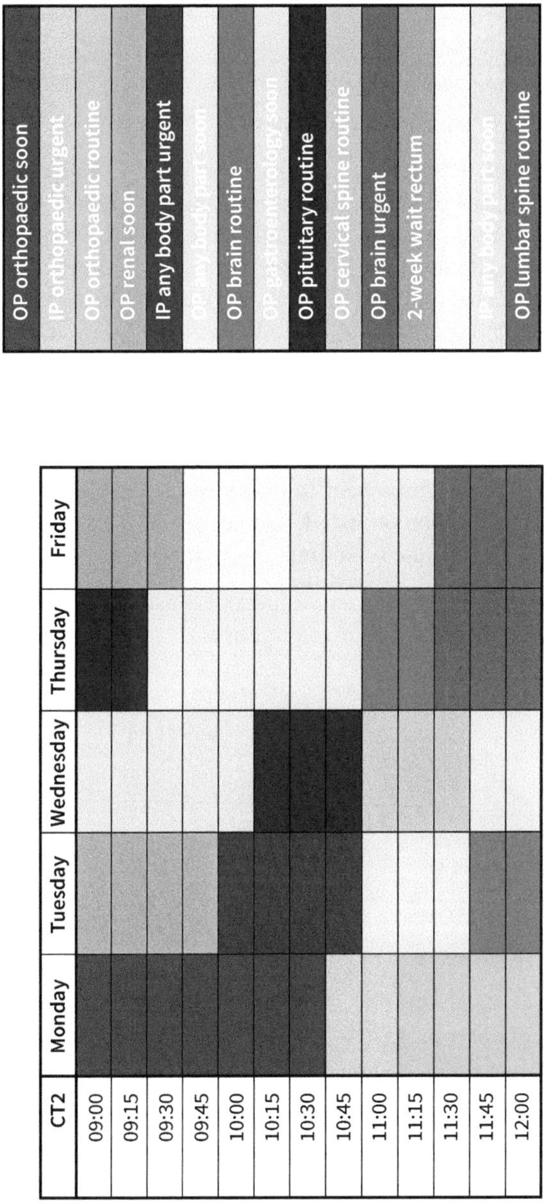

Figure 10.12 Example of carve-out of CT appointment slots. OP, outpatient.

CT2	Monday	Tuesday	Wednesday	Thursday	Friday
09:00					
09:15					
09:30					
09:45					
10:00					
10:15					
10:30					
10:45					
11:00					
11:15					
11:30					
11:45					
12:00					

Legend:
- OP orthopaedic soon
- IP orthopaedic urgent
- OP orthopaedic routine
- OP renal soon
- IP any body part urgent
- OP any body part soon
- OP brain routine
- OP gastroenterology soon
- OP pituitary routine
- OP cervical spine routine
- OP brain urgent
- 2-week wait rectum
- IP any body part soon
- OP lumbar spine routine

STRATEGIES FOR TESTING CHANGES AND PDSA CYCLES

Once the maps and measures have been produced and the causes of poor flow are identified, the next step is to test changes in a controlled manner, remembering that all processes should be measured before and after the test of change. If the test of change has a positive impact, it can be accelerated; if the test of change has a negative impact, it can be quickly stopped or amended. A plan, do, study, act (PDSA) cycle can be used to test an idea on a small scale; then monitor the impact before implementing a wide-scale change (**Figure 10.13**). However, adapting the approach to 'study' first, rather than 'plan', ensures that the team have studied what the maps and measures are demonstrating. As we would do with a patient, it is important to diagnose the problem first, then plan what needs to be done or tested.

The following needs to be done to address the changes:

■ Remove any steps that do not add any value and consider the wider pathway and the upstream or downstream impact.

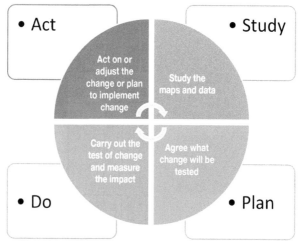

Figure 10.13 Adapted PDSA cycle.

- Reduce the number of hand-offs: every time there is a hand-off, there is the potential for duplications, errors and delays.
- Reduce or eliminate batching because it creates delays in a process, as previously discussed.
- Reduce the (carve-out) number of queues by pooling lists and removing appointments allocated for specific priorities, exams, sources or consultants.
- Reduce delays at the bottleneck. Visible observations and maps will demonstrate where the bottleneck is, such as registering at the reception.
- Undertake steps that can be done outside the room before the patient enters the room, such as cannulation before the patient enters the clinical room, to ensure that the equipment does not become an expensive phlebotomy couch. This will reduce the cycle times.
- Plan medical imaging and radiotherapy appointments to suit the patient and mutually agree the appointment to reduce failure to attend (DNA) and cancellations. Consider combining multiple appointments or linking the appointment to the patient's next outpatient visit when possible.
- Adopt a 'first-in, first-out' (FIFO) or 'by due date appointment' order for booking and reporting to reduce variation.
- Review skill mix and ensure staff are working to the 'top of their licence'. Ensure registered professionals are not undertaking tasks suitable for support staff, for example allocating appointments, cannulation, moving patients into the room, positioning for imaging or treatment.
- Equally, role extension for radiographers can include reporting and undertaking interventional examinations, which will reduce the workload on radiologists.

Once changes have been tested, measure the impact of the change, and repeat, as some changes take longer to have an impact. Keep comparing against the baseline measure. Agree and communicate the changes to ensure sustainability and to reduce the chances of a member of staff who has not been informed of the new process reversing the change. Good visual management using written standard operating procedures (SOPs), photos of trolley layout, improvement notice boards and daily huddles are great ways to reinforce new processes.

DATA FOR BASELINES AND MONITORING

There are several data sets that are monitored nationally by the NHS, and baselining sites where you can compare your performance against that of your peers. The following are specific to England. The other UK nations will have their own specific targets and priorities.

DM01

The monthly diagnostics waiting times and activity return[5] collects data on waiting times and activity for 15 key diagnostic tests and procedures, including:

- MRI;
- CT;
- non-obstetric ultrasound;
- dual-energy X-ray absorptiometry (DEXA) scanning, also commonly referred to as DXA scanning.

It contains aggregate-level data submitted by providers and is measured against the 6-week outpatient target in line with the NHS constitution. NHS England published new guidance in May 2021 for the prioritisation of waiting lists for diagnostic procedures. The results are published nationally on the NHS website.[5]

Diagnostic Imaging Dataset

The Diagnostic Imaging Dataset (DID)[6] is a central collection of detailed information about diagnostic imaging tests carried out on NHS patients, extracted from the local RIS and submitted monthly. These data capture information about the following:

- referral source;

- patient type;
- details of the test (type of test and body site);
- demographic information, such as:
  - registered general practice;
  - patient postcode;
  - ethnicity;
  - gender;
  - date of birth;
- waiting times for each diagnostic imaging event, from time of test request to time of reporting.

NHS Digital collects the data at the patient level. It is reported in summary form as official statistics.

Model Health System

The Model Health System (formerly the Model Hospital)[11] is a data-driven improvement tool that supports health and care systems to improve their productivity, efficiency, patient outcomes and population health. It provides benchmarked insights across the quality of care, productivity and organisational culture to identify opportunities for improvement.

Data for Performance

NHS England and the Department of Health and Social Care have made a series of pledges, which are set out in the NHS constitution. These cover a range of measures for different aspects of healthcare; some will impact on Medical Imaging and Radiotherapy Departments.

Emergency Department Operational Targets

These targets relate to the time it takes for a patient to be discharged, transferred or admitted when they attend the ED, and are often referred to as 'the 4-hour target'. The latest target, set out in the 2024/25 priorities and operational planning guidance, is that 78% of patients must be seen within 4 hours of attending the ED.[12]

Cancer 2-Week Wait

An urgent 2-week referral means that a patient will be offered an appointment with a hospital specialist within 2 weeks of a GP referral; this includes medical imaging tests.

Faster Diagnosis Target of 28 Days

NHS England has introduced a new target called the Faster Diagnosis Standard (FDS). The target is that a patient should not wait more than 28 days from referral to finding out whether or not they have a cancer.

6-Week Outpatient Targets

The diagnostic operational standard stipulates that less than 1% of patients should wait more than 6 weeks for a diagnostic test. This is measured monthly via the DM01.

18-Week Rule

The maximum waiting time for a non-urgent, consultant-led treatment, including diagnostic tests, is 18 weeks from the day an appointment is booked through the NHS referral service, or when the hospital receives a referral letter.

CHAPTER SUMMARY

- To deliver highly effective and efficient services, it is important to understand the factors that influence the flow of patients through the patient pathway.
- Continuous quality improvement (CQI) is used by teams and organisations to make changes by continuously adapting and refining processes.
- Be clear on the improvement focus; define the scope.
- Developing the correct strategy prior to any improvement effort is key to success.
- Many problems associated with poor flow are caused by poor processes.

- Walk the pathway of the patient.
- Mapping allows the detailed pathway to be documented and visualised.
- Establish a baseline of measures (i.e. referrals, activity, backlog, lead times and cycle times) to diagnose the problem.
- Once the maps and measures have been produced and the causes of poor flow are identified, the next step is to test changes in a controlled manner.
- Reducing variation will improve patient flow.
- Policy constraints (time traps, batching and carve-out) are assumptions and beliefs that have been introduced to try and improve a process, but, unwittingly, can make the lead times longer and will create variation.
- If the average demand equals the average activity, then the waiting list will stay constant.
- Remeasure after a test of change and remeasure to monitor changes.

FURTHER READING

- NHS England. Statistical Process Control Tool. Available at www.england.nhs.uk/statistical-process-control-tool/.

REFERENCES

1. NHS England. Transforming Imaging Services in England: A National Strategy for Imaging. 2019. Available at www.england.nhs.uk/transforming-imaging-services-in-england/.
2. Richards, M. Diagnostics: Recovery and Renewal – Report of the Independent Review of Diagnostic Services for NHS England. 2020. Available at www.england.nhs.uk/publication/diagnostics-recovery-and-renewal-report-of-the-independent-review-of-diagnostic-services-for-nhs-england/.
3. NHS England. Radiology: GIRFT Programme National Specialty Report. 2020. Available at https://gettingitrightfirsttime.co.uk/medical_specialties/radiology/.

4. NHS England. 2023/24 Priorities and Operational Planning Guidance. 2022. Available at www.england.nhs.uk/publication/2023-24-priorities-and-operational-planning-guidance/.

5. NHS England. Monthly Diagnostic Waiting Times and Activity. Available at www.england.nhs.uk/statistics/statistical-work-areas/diagnostics-waiting-times-and-activity/monthly-diagnostics-waiting-times-and-activity.

6. NHS England. Diagnostic Imaging Dataset. Available at www.england.nhs.uk/statistics/statistical-work-areas/diagnostic-imaging-dataset/.

7. Westwood, N., James-Moore, M. and Cook, M. Going Lean in the NHS. NHS Institute for Innovation and Improvement. 2017. Available at www.england.nhs.uk/improvement-hub/wp-content/uploads/sites/44/2017/11/Going-Lean-in-the-NHS.pdf.

8. Heathcare Systems Engineering. Available at www.improvement-science.co.uk.

9. NHS IMPACT. Available at www.england.nhs.uk/nhsimpact/.

10. Kübler-Ross, E. and Kessler, D. *On Grief and Grieving*. London: Simon & Schuster UK; 2014.

11. NHS England. The Model Health System: Available at www.england.nhs.uk/applications/model-hospital/.

12. NHS England. 2024/25 Priorities and Operational Planning Guidance. Available at www.england.nhs.uk/wp-content/uploads/2024/03/PRN00715-2024-25-priorities-and-operational-planning-guidance-27.03.2024.pdf.

11. SERVICE USER INVOLVEMENT

Amanda Martin and Louise Kemp

INTRODUCTION

Before exploring the concept of service user involvement, it is important to address the differing terminology. Some professions prefer to use the term '**patient**', while others will use the term '**client**' or '**customer**'. The UK Health and Care Professions Council (HCPC) uses the term '**service user**' to encompass all those who access healthcare, and so this phrase will be used throughout this chapter.[1]

The value of involving service users is immense and there are many reports of its positive impact,[2,3] including improvement in safety and quality of healthcare provision, increased accessibility to services and enrichment in healthcare education programmes.[4,5] However, it does not come without its challenges. Appropriate involvement takes time and resources and is often a low priority in a busy department that sees service user involvement as simply the collection of feedback. Smiley-face surveys, with emojis indicating level of satisfaction, are quick and simple to administer, but the data are not particularly meaningful. These are useful for compiling general satisfaction levels, but may give false confidence, or are not specific enough to be able to inform change. The value of soliciting feedback comes from seeing the service through the eyes of the servicer user. This may be achieved only through direct involvement. However, some service users may be reluctant to be involved due to lack of confidence, the use of technical language or the power imbalance between service user and healthcare professional. Additionally, some sections of society may be under-represented due to age or illness, for example, so their views may not be captured.

DOI: 9781003380078-11

Staff may be uncomfortable with service users making decisions about their service, but it must be remembered that the service user is the one experiencing and seeing the problems that staff are often oblivious to. These challenges are likely to be the cause of the numerous reports of dissatisfaction and the disparaging external quality reports that often judge healthcare provision to be inadequate.

User feedback serves as an important quality measure for the department and should ideally be built into local governance/performance and key performance indicators (KPIs) to ensure it remains high on the quality agenda.

CONCEPTS OF SERVICE USER INVOLVEMENT

Numerous phrases are used when discussing the engagement or involvement of service users, some focused on the patient as an individual and the care that they receive, and others on a collective group of individuals experiencing that service.

Service user involvement from an individual's perspective is about their individual needs being met. This is often referred to as **personalised care**, **person-centred care**, **patient-centred care** or **values-based care**. The service user is involved in their own personal care by being provided with the information and support to enable them to make decisions about their care pathway. This can range from a simple decision about a specific treatment to more complex decisions about long-term care pathways. They are subsequently more likely to engage and be compliant with treatment plans if they are choosing what matters to them. They will be able to manage their own health and wellbeing and are less likely to require formal medical input, thus reducing the number of hospital attendances, the number of admissions and instances of associated possible complications of hospital stays, such as hospital-acquired infections.

In 2018, and in response to the NHS Five Year Forward View,[6] the UK Society of Radiographers (SoR) published a set of guiding principles outlining values that are important to the patient in a number of different domains, including service development and delivery, education and research. In the service development domain, the principles are associated with the involvement of service users and experts from, for example, peer groups in the design/redesign of services. This builds on the World Health Organization (WHO) document on **integrated people-centred care**, which focuses on the need to develop services based on the needs of people.[7] NHS England supports this approach and has developed a strategy for involving service users, focusing on when and how to involve them.[8]

This chapter will focus on the wider concept of service user involvement for the purpose of improving a current service or designing a new service. It will start by briefly exploring the methods of receiving patient feedback before looking at the different ways in which service users can be involved, before finally outlining a complaints management process in order to learn valuable lessons from patient experiences.

RECEIVING FEEDBACK FROM SERVICE USERS

Service users may be invited by the organisation to give feedback in numerous ways:

- via text messaging systems;
- by filling in paper forms at the time of the visit;
- through digital surveys on a tablet or kiosk located in the department.

Some departments have recruited 'secret shoppers' from their service users to provide more specific and detailed feedback on their experiences. This involves a service user gathering particular information about the quality of care that they receive. Shadowing a service user will also enable valuable information to be gathered through observational study, which can further be expanded on through later discussion with the service user. Involving service users in a 'walk-through' of a service can be very effective in evaluating the service's approach, such as experiencing it from the viewpoint of service users with specific needs, for example autism or dementia, or of specific sections of society, for example children. Feedback may also be collected at organisational level, for example via the **NHS Friends and Family Test** (FFT) in the UK.[9] This is a simple questionnaire, delivered in a paper format, via text message, via telephone call or through a website. It is designed to help those who provide healthcare services to understand the level of satisfaction a patient has with the service and to identify where improvements are needed. It is, however, recognised that the level of qualitative data that are actionable is limited,[10] and it can be difficult to identify service-specific information in this way, particularly if a visit involves multiple departments. Nevertheless, there are often themes within this broader feedback that could apply to any department, and these can be incorporated into quality improvement activities and quality metrics. Alternatively, service users may proactively offer feedback by contacting the organisation's **Patient Advice and Liaison Service** (PALS), by telling the **Care Quality Commission** (CQC) about their experience or by leaving a review on the NHS services website or other online review forums.

Feedback may present as positive or negative comments. Leaders should pay attention to the things that service users respond well to, as well as those issues identified that, when remedied, will improve the service. Communicating improvements to the users of the service, for example in 'you said, we did' posters, demonstrates that the service is listening and can encourage service users to provide feedback with the confidence that their responses will be acted upon.

HOW TO INVOLVE SERVICE USERS

The drive to include service users in everything we do has increased in the 21st century, with many encouraging, supporting and even legislating for this.[11] One of the core principles outlined in the NHS Constitution for England is that '**the patient will be at the heart of everything the NHS does**'.[12] The NHS Long Term Plan[13] is built on the concept introduced in the NHS Five Year Forward View[6] that service users should hold the power in deciding on their care and the way that services are delivered. In addition, the SoR response to the NHS Five Year Forward View was to publish a document 'Patient Public and Practitioner Partnerships within Imaging and Radiotherapy', which also advocates involving service users in the development of services.[14] It urges practitioners to listen to the voice of the service user and to understand their experiences in their words so that their needs and values are embedded into the services that are provided. The service user voice can be heard through many channels:

- analysing and acting on feedback, which may be received through complaints, incidents, questionnaires or focus groups;
- service user representatives within formal meeting structures, for example a representative on a divisional governance board;
- their involvement in the development of service user information;
- their involvement in planning and development meetings for new or reviewed services;
- provision of insights to help inform policy and in setting standards;
- in the design and delivery of education and research towards person-centred care;
- in the recruitment and selection of staff.

Feedback from and direct involvement of service users is essential in understanding what it feels like to be a user within the service, what the quality of care is like and what is important to the people experiencing care within the service. They will have a unique insight, which may shape the future of the service in which they are involved. Understanding their experience and keeping their voice at the centre of everything we do serves a number of purposes:

- highlights areas for improvement;
- provides evidence to support improvement initiatives, for example in business cases;
- shapes service design or redesign;
- monitors the effectiveness of service improvements or changes in patient experience;
- supports staff engagement through sharing positive feedback;
- informs the CQC inspection 'key lines of enquiry' (KLOEs) by demonstrating how patient feedback is listened to and addressed.[15]

The service user may be acting as an individual representing their own views, and sometimes referred to as the '**expert patient**', or they may be representing the views of a wider group of service users, usually from a **user group**. Regardless of how the voice of the user is heard, the experience behind that voice should be used to benefit service users of the future, resulting in a person-centred service. In addition, having service users on development groups may focus the minds and attitudes of the staff, as they are likely to be challenged about what they see as the only way to deliver the service.

Involving service users in the planning and delivery of services ranges from simply providing them with information to enabling them to influence decisions by using that information appropriately. This is called the **ladder of engagement and participation**, with each 'rung' on the ladder being a different level of involvement (**Table 11.1**).[16] The aim is not to reach the top of the ladder, with full control for the service user on all occasions, but to use the 'rung' that is relevant to the situation.

Table 11.1 Example of a ladder of user participation.

Level	Service user engagement
Level 1	Provision of information through leaflets or posters. No formal engagement or discussion with a view to influencing change.
Level 2	Seeking service user views through questionnaires, feedback forms or interviews. These views may or may not be considered when decisions are being made.
Level 3	Views expressed by service users are considered when making decisions. Their views have a direct impact on how a service may be developed.
Level 4	Service users are involved in the meetings and workshops and are able to influence the outcome of any discussions.
Level 5	Decisions are made by the service user.

MANAGING FEEDBACK FROM COMPLAINTS

Valuable feedback may be received through the complaints process. This should not be seen in a negative way. Indeed, it can be seen in a positive way, as this is feedback that a patient has not been asked to supply, and often encompasses meaningful data. It is often the opportunity to stop and review the service from a user's point of view, with a service user who may be willing to be involved in the improvement process. Management of the complaints process is key to utilising this opportunity to improve. It should be done to facilitate learning and drive improvements, rather than to apportion blame.

In the UK health system, 225,570 complaints were made in 2021/22.[17] Although only 26.8% were upheld, every complaint must be seen as an opportunity for improvement based on feedback from a service user. According to NHS Resolution, a complaint is 'an expression of dissatisfaction that requires a response',[18] and can be made several ways:

- verbally to a staff member;
- in writing, either as a letter or a feedback form response;
- electronically via email;
- through social media forums or websites such as Care Opinion;
- through a Member of Parliament (MP);
- through the parliamentary and health service ombudsman;
- through the HCPC;
- through the CQC.

Complaints can be made by the patient; by a person who is impacted by a decision made, for example a relative or carer; or by a representative of the patient if the patient lacks capacity or is deceased. If the complaint is not made by the patient, then consent to discuss the circumstances around the complaint may be required from the patient, if possible.

Complaints are categorised as **informal** and **formal**, and both can be made in all the above ways. However, if a formal investigation and a formal response is required, this generally initiates the formal complaints process and the patient, carer or their representative should be encouraged to put the complaint in writing, if it isn't already. An informal complaint is better managed at the time that it is made, either by the person receiving the complaint or by a more senior staff member. It is important to seek clarity on the complaint and to ask the complainant if they want to be informed of the outcome. Many informal complainants simply want to know that somebody is acting on their concerns, but some will want to know what the outcome is, and the action taken.

This should be communicated with them as soon as possible, or within 2 days after the complaint is made.[18] Keeping a record of informal complaints will allow trends to be identified, allow improvement projects to be planned and ensure that positive change is taking place as a result of this feedback. Occasionally, an informal complaint cannot be resolved; the complainant should be advised about making a formal complaint so that a full investigation can take place.

A formal complaint investigation will take time; however, it is good practice to acknowledge the complaint within 3 days of receiving it, either verbally or in writing, with an outline of the complaints process and what can be expected going forward. All formal complaints, whether verbal or in writing, must be logged with the department that specifically deals with service user experience and complaints. While there is no formal national timescale for a final response, local policy or commissioning bodies may specify timescales. It is again good practice to investigate, respond and close complaints in a timely manner, generally within 6 months, as the cause of the complaint may need eliminating, minimising or adapting to reduce the chance of future complaints or incidents. Throughout the process, communication with the complainant must remain open and honest and their voice must be listened to. The final response will need the input of the appropriate specialty senior leader, but it is sent by the '**responsible person**', which is the person who is responsible for ensuring compliance with the Local Authority Social Services and National Health Service Complaints (England) Regulations 2009.[19] This is likely to be the chief executive officer (CEO). An improvement plan should be developed after every complaint that addresses the points raised, the actions to address them, the timescales and the person responsible for completing the action. This should be reviewed regularly to make sure that improvements are being made.

If a complaint involves a concerning attitude or behaviours of a regulated health professional, the regulatory body may be informed, and they may decide to commence a fitness to practise investigation. This is not simply about the competence of an individual, but it also involves their character and their ability to carry out their role in relation to their health. The panel investigating the complaint will decide whether there is a case to answer and, if so, it will be directed to the appropriate fitness to practise committee, after which the decision will be made on the future of the registrant.

CHAPTER SUMMARY

- The value of involving service users is immense; however, it does come with challenges.
- Appropriate involvement takes time and resources in order to collect data that are actionable.
- Concepts of service user involvement range from their involvement in their own individual care to the involvement in wider healthcare practices associated with service design.
- User feedback is an important quality measure.
- Feedback can be gathered through numerous methods, and both negative and positive feedback should support improvement.
- Service users can be involved in many aspects of healthcare, and can range from their involvement in the provision of information to them making decisions about a service.
- Valuable feedback is received through the complaints process, and it is important to view any complaint as a positive step in improving the service.

FURTHER READING

- NHS England and NHS Improvement. Online Library of Quality, Service Improvement and Redesign Tools: Gaining Insights from Working in Partnership with Health Service Users. 2022. Available at https://aqua.nhs.uk/wp-content/uploads/2023/07/qsir-gaining-insights.pdf.

REFERENCES

1. HCPC. Service User and Carer Involvement. 2018. Available at www.hcpc-uk.org/education/resources/education-standards/service-user-and-carer-involvement/.

2. Smith, S., Abbas, M. and Zegarra, A. Overcoming challenges in service user involvement in an older people's mental health service. *Mental Health and Social Inclusion* 2020:**24**(3):151–155.

3. WHO. Technical Series on Safer Primary Care: Patient Engagement. 2016. Available at www.who.int/publications/i/item/9789241511629.

4. Omeni, E., Barnes, M., MacDonald, D., Crawford, M. and Rose, D. Service user involvement: impact and participation: a survey of service user and staff perspectives. *BMC Health Services Research* 2014;**14**:491.

5. Gordon, M., Gupta, S., Thornton, D., Reid, M., Mallen, E. and Melling, A. Patient/service user involvement in medical education: a best evidence medical education (BEME) systematic review: BEME Guide No. 58. *Medical Teacher* 2019;**42**(1):4–16.

6. NHS England. Five Year Forward View. 2014. Available at www.england.nhs.uk/publication/nhs-five-year-forward-view/.

7. WHO. Integrated People-Centred Care. 2016. Available at www.who.int/health-topics/integrated-people-centered-care.

8. NHS England and NHS Improvement. Online Library of Quality, Service Improvement and Redesign Tools: Gaining Insights from/ Working in Partnership with Health Service Users. Available at https://aqua.nhs.uk/wp-content/uploads/2023/07/qsir-gaining-insights.pdf.

9. NHS. Friends and Family Test. Available at www.nhs.uk/using-the-nhs/about-the-nhs/friends-and-family-test-fft/.

10. Skillen, J.D. The Friends and Family Test: from card sorts to control charts. *Methodological Innovations* 2019;**12**(2).

11. Francis, R. Report of the Mid Staffordshire NHS Trust Public Inquiry: Executive Summary. 2013. Available at https://assets.publishing.service.gov.uk/media/5a7ba0faed915d13110607c8/0947.pdf.

12. NHS. NHS Constitution for England. 2012. Available at www.gov.uk/government/publications/the-nhs-constitution-for-england.

13. NHS. The NHS Long Term Plan. 2019. Available at www.longtermplan.nhs.uk/wp-content/uploads/2019/08/nhs-long-term-plan-version-1.2.pdf.

14. SoR. *Patient Public and Practitioner Partnerships within Imaging and Radiotherapy: Guiding Principles.* London: SoR; 2018.

15. CQC. Key Lines of Enquiry for Healthcare Services. 2022. Available at www.cqc.org.uk/guidance-providers/healthcare/key-lines-enquiry-healthcare-services.

16. Arnstein, S.R. A ladder of citizen participation. *Journal of the American Planning Association* 1969;**35**(4):216–224.

17. NHS Digital. Data on Written Complaints in the NHS, 2021–22. 2022. Available at https://digital.nhs.uk/data-and-information/publications/statistical/data-on-written-complaints-in-the-nhs/2021-22.

18. NHS Resolution. Complaints Policy. 2019. Available at https://resolution.nhs.uk/wp-content/uploads/2021/03/CG12-Complaints-Policy.pdf.

19. Local Authority Social Services and National Health Service Complaints (England) Regulations 2009. Available at www.legislation.gov.uk/uksi/2009/309/made?view=plain.

12. RESEARCH, CLINICAL AUDIT AND SERVICE EVALUATION IN PRACTICE

Amanda Martin, Jo Cresswell and Peter Hogg

INTRODUCTION

Research improves therapy outcomes, advances diagnostic potential and enhances patient wellbeing. Research is also used to define and evaluate radiographer roles; without it, advanced and consultant radiographer practice would not exist in the UK. A medical imaging or radiotherapy department with a good research culture, and which participates in interdisciplinary research, supports improved care, supports research projects that are more relevant to patients and provides opportunities for patients to be involved in high-quality clinical trials.[1]

It is important to distinguish between research, service evaluations and clinical audits.

- Research is a rigorous systematic study that results in new knowledge. Research outcomes can have local, national and global value.
- A service evaluation is a method for determining the quality of the service that is being delivered and is valuable only to that service.[2] The results are often used to inform local decision-making for the purposes of service improvement.
- A clinical audit is the systematic investigation of a part of the, or the whole, clinical service to determine if it meets the required standard. It is usually associated with a quality improvement cycle, in which actions are taken to improve care.

DOI: 9781003380078-12

Table 12.1 Simple examples of how service evaluations, clinical audits and research can be used in healthcare settings.

Service evaluation	Undertake evaluation to identify how well the general practice chest imaging service is performing in relation to, for example, appointment wait times, report turnaround times or quality of reports.
Clinical audit	Undertake audit to measure the reporting turnaround times for the computed tomography (CT) stroke service against best-practice standards.
Research	Undertake research to identify the most effective way of delivering a new interventional procedure.

Together, research, service evaluations and clinical audits aim to improve patient care and wellbeing. **Table 12.1** gives simple indications of how service evaluations, clinical audits and research can be used in the clinical setting.

To meet professional standards and patient expectations, radiography must be evidence-based.[3] All radiographers must use evidence in their practice, examples of which include research findings, audit results and service evaluation outcomes. Consequently, all radiographers should be competent at searching and critiquing peer-reviewed literature and other types of published information. By contrast, only some radiographers will conduct research; this will be instigated by needs and the available resources. Unsurprisingly, due to limited human and physical resources, decisions need to be made regarding what research, service evaluation and clinical audit will be done. Such decisions should align with strategic priorities, which could be local and/or national.

SERVICE EVALUATION

A service evaluation is about reviewing a service and judging how well it is doing by scrutinising processes and outcomes. It determines whether the service outcomes are being met and is useful during and following a change to a service.[4] There is no specific standard to measure against. For clarity, a service may consist of multiple standards that come together to achieve the required outcome. An evaluation is focused on that overall outcome rather than on the individual standards within it. A service evaluation should result in plans for driving service improvement and/or service redesign.

A service evaluation can be either formative or summative.[4] A **formative evaluation** is employed throughout the development and implementation of a new service or as changes are being made to an established service, with a view to modifying the changes to ensure that the required outcome is achieved.[5] A **summative evaluation** focuses on an established service to identify how well it is doing in meeting the required outcome. It may be used to assure commissioners that money is being well spent,[6] to inform clinical guidelines or as a baseline audit where audit standards are set.

Prior to undertaking a service evaluation, it is important to understand the question that is being asked so that the correct information can be gathered. This involves working in partnership with stakeholders. Partnership working helps with designing the evaluation method and ensures that the correct information is gathered. There are several ways to gather information, depending on what is being evaluated.

- *Questionnaires and interviews.* These can be structured, semi-structured or unstructured, and aim to assess a range of topics from satisfaction to experience of care. Satisfaction, which is a measure of whether expectations have been met, is often directly related to quality.[7]
- *Direct observation.* Specific aspects of the actions of staff or patients are documented, such as interactions with others, time to complete tasks or movement between different locations. This may lead to process mapping (see Chapter 10).
- *Extracting information from clinical databases.* A retrospective process involving the extraction of existing data, which is faster than prospective collection as the data have already been recorded. Its limitations include the following: missing/inaccurate data, the data might not give a direct measure of what is being investigated and they may not be reflective of current practice, depending on the timescales set for data collection.

CLINICAL AUDITS

There can be numerous reasons for conducting a clinical audit, for example:

- to check standards of care;
- to check compliance with local or national policies, procedures or directives;
- following a complaint or an incident to assess the extent of the problem.

The aim of a clinical audit is to systematically measure current practice against **predetermined standards** and identify improvements. Standards can be locally, regionally or nationally set. An example of a national standard in radiology is the following: the UK National Institute for Health and Care Excellence (NICE)[8] states that an acute stroke patient should undergo a CT scan in 'the next available slot and definitely within 1 hour'. This will define the data that are required; for example, in relation to this standard, data associated with a measure of time are needed. Data can be collected several ways, but only data that will determine if practice complies with the standard must be collected. Data can be collected **prospectively** or **retrospectively**; each method has advantages and disadvantages. Prospective data collection allows data to be validated as the collection is in progress, but could be flawed if staff change their practice because of a concurrent audit. Retrospective data collection may result in a more accurate reflection of practice. Although it is reviewing practices that have already occurred, it can be concluded that it is reflective of current practice. It can, however, be time-consuming unless it can be done electronically through a computer database such as a radiology information system or patient management system.

A suitable **data collection tool** will be needed. It may be useful to pilot it by completing one or two data sets so that any errors are identified early in the process and can be corrected prior to completion of the audit.

Depending on the number of data available, a suitable **sample size** may need to be set in order to not be overwhelmed by the number of data. The number within the sample needs to be manageable, yet representative of the practice being assessed. No formal calculation methods are available for service evaluations and clinical audits, unlike research; an example of a method to calculate a 'research' sample size can be found online at *www.calculator.net/sample-size-calculator.html*.

Unlike with research using a quantitative method, a statistical approach is unlikely to be needed in the case of an audit. Sample selection should be determined by the audit population. If this has not changed (retrospective data collection) or is not likely to change (prospective data collection) through the period of audit, then **random sampling** can be used. If the population could change, then a predetermined time frame is set, for example, every patient attending in a 2-month period will be included. Make sure that **bias** is not introduced and that a broad range of practice is included in the sample size by covering all days and all shift patterns. It may also be necessary to identify inclusion and exclusion criteria. **Rapid cycle sampling** allows for a small sample size to be assessed so that results can be achieved quickly, and any problems identified and managed in a timely manner. This also enables a faster turnaround of improvement and re-audit.

Once data have been collected and analysed, if the standard is not being met, then an **action plan** is needed that includes an indication of what needs to be changed, an outline of how this is to be done and identification of the individuals involved and the time frame in which it is to be completed. Any changes must be implemented, and the audit repeated. As such, audit is a continuous cycle and not a 'one-off' exercise (**Figure 12.1**).

For further information on audits, please refer to the Healthcare Quality Improvement Partnership (HQIP) document Best Practice in Clinical Audit.[9]

RESEARCH

Radiography is an applied field and because of this radiography research should really focus on outcomes that have practical value. Contemporary radiography research tends to address complex problems that are frequently transnational, multifaceted and multilayered.[10]

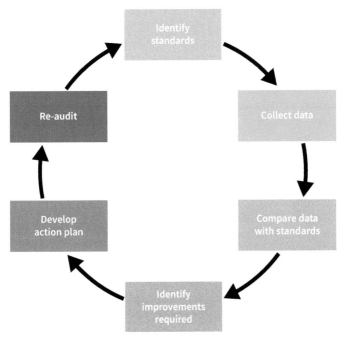

Figure 12.1 The audit cycle.

To investigate such problems, teams must possess the right skill, disciplinary and, as required, multinational mix. Within such teams, radiographers may play a range of roles, including providing the clinician's/educator's viewpoint and conducting the research. For the former, it is important that radiographers are included at the outset as this will facilitate the translation of research findings into practice. For the latter, the radiographer must be a competent researcher and various training schemes must exist. The basic training for a researcher is **Doctor of Philosophy** (PhD); this takes 3 years to complete (full-time), but, beyond that point, the radiographer will need a further 5–10 years of experience and supervised development to become a competent researcher/research lead. Aside from a PhD, a wide range of **continuing professional development** (CPD) research training opportunities exist at different levels; these are often available in-house, provided by external organisations and offered to multi-professional audiences. Radiographers can access research training funding to support, for example, their PhD; a good source of this is the **National Institute for Health and Care Research** (NIHR).[11] Universities often provide practical support for radiographers to make funding applications for PhD and other research training opportunities, as can healthcare organisations.

Research is time-consuming and can require expensive physical resources. Funding is therefore needed, and grant applications must be made by research teams to meet costs. Many grant funding organisations exist, offering a few thousand to several million pounds per project. Funding is allocated on a competitive basis, and it can take up to a year to write a grant application and to know the outcome. Most grant funding bodies are oversubscribed, and typically only about 20% of applications are successful. Grant writing is complex and time-consuming, but it is within the capability of a competent researcher. Most large healthcare organisations and universities have central research support services that can help in grant writing.

At this stage it is worth noting that, while a growing number of radiographers possess a doctoral qualification, very few are competent researchers. This is because many who possess a doctoral qualification have not developed adequately as a researcher beyond acquiring the PhD qualification – this can generally happen only when the radiographer is an integral part of an active research group or research-intensive department. It is therefore important to determine if the people who are to conduct research have the right competencies, support and mentoring to do so, which may not be inferred from possession of a PhD alone.

For radiography research to be beneficial, it must be used in practice. For this to occur, the research team should take steps, in partnership with the community the research serves, to embed research outcomes into practice. A key step in this translation process is dissemination of research findings; the traditional way of doing this is through peer-reviewed journal articles. Networks are also an important way to disseminate and embed research findings. There is increasing emphasis on researchers to evidence real-world impact from research, and on universities, clinical practitioners and patient groups to evidence, evaluate and disseminate this research. Papers presented at seminars and conferences help the dissemination process, but tend to reach smaller audiences than journal articles, and the peer-review quality assurance is lower than that associated with journal publications. Textbooks might play a part in dissemination; however, radiography books tend to bring together information that has been available in journals for many years. Books may also contain elements of practice that have not been subjected to the rigours of research.

Ethics, Consent and Confidentiality

Ethics processes exist to protect research participants from poor practice and harm. Processes and standards are based on the **Helsinki Declaration**.[12] Ethics committees exist to ensure compliance with good ethical principles, and they receive written applications from research teams. **Ethics committees** therefore decide whether or not a project can go ahead. Deciding which ethics committee to seek approval from can be complex, but, usually, an NHS committee might need to give approval if NHS patients are to be involved in a research study.[13] A competent researcher should know which committee needs to give permission and how to write the ethics application. Ethics committees tend to span across institutions and are thus not specific to a particular organisation. For clinical audits and service evaluations, there is no need to ask permission from an ethics committee. Instead, processes and committees exist within organisations to vet and approve audits and evaluations before they go ahead.

When people, including patients and healthcare workers, are to become involved with research, an audit or an evaluation as participants, they should normally give their **consent**. To do this they should be adequately informed about what is being asked of them and adequate details of the study should be given to them; this is termed '**informed consent**'.[14] We have purposefully used the word 'normally', as there are certain types of study in which the research participants do not know they are the subject of a study and will therefore not give consent. Such studies need special consideration and will not be considered in this chapter.

Confidentiality and **data protection** should be considered when conducting research, service evaluations and clinical audits. These topics are considered in Chapter 16.

Further Reading about Research

Thousands of books have been published about research methods and statistics. Most of these are generic in nature and are thus applicable to radiographers working in medical imaging and radiotherapy; we encourage you to use this invaluable and extensive resource. Because there are so many published books on research methods and statistics, very few have needed to be written specifically for medical imaging and radiotherapy. However, some do exist and below are two that we recommend:

- Seeram, E., Davidson, R., England, A. and McEntee, M.F. *Research for Medical Imaging and Radiation Sciences.* Cham: Springer; 2022.
- Ramlaul, A. *Medical Imaging and Radiotherapy Research: Skills and Strategies.* Second edition. Cham: Springer; 2020.

CHAPTER SUMMARY

- Research, clinical audit and service evaluation aim to improve patient care and wellbeing.
- Research is a rigorous systematic study that results in new knowledge.
- Service evaluation is a method for determining the quality of the service that is being delivered and is valuable only to that service.
- Clinical audit is the systematic investigation of a part of the, or the whole, clinical service to determine if it meets the required standard.
- Ethics processes exist to protect research participants from poor practice and harm.
- Ethics approval is needed if patients are involved in research studies, but not for service evaluations or clinical audits.

REFERENCES

1. Selby, P., Popescu, R., Lawler, M., Butcher, H. and Costa, A. Future developments of multidisciplinary team cancer care. *American Society of Clinical Oncology Educational Book* 2019;**39**:332–340.

2. NHS. Research, Service Evaluation or Audit? Available at https://nspccro.nihr.ac.uk/working-with-us/research-service-evaluation-or-audit.

3. College of Radiographers. 2021–2026 Research Strategy. 2021. Available at www.collegeofradiographcrs.ac.uk/getattachment/Research-grants-and-funding/cor-research-strategy/cor-research-strategy-2021-26.pdf?lang=en-GB.

4. The Health Foundation. Evaluation: What to Consider. 2015. Available at www.health.org.uk/publications/evaluation-what-to-consider.

5. Moule, P., Armoogum, J., Dodd, E. and Donskey, A. Practical guidance on undertaking a service evaluation. *Nursing Standard* 2016;**30**(45):46–51.

6. Health and Social Care Act 2012. Available at www.legislation.gov.uk/ukpga/2012/7/contents.

7. Aiken, L.H., Sloane, D.M., Ball, J., Bruyneel, L., Rafferty, A.M. and Griffiths, P. Patient satisfaction with hospital care and nurses in England: an observational study. *BMJ Open* 2021;**8**:e019189.

8. NICE. *Stroke and Transient Ischaemic Attack in Over 16s: Diagnosis and Initial Management.* NG128. London: NICE; 2019.

9. HQIP. Best Practice in Clinical Audit. 2020. Available at www.hqip.org.uk/resource/best-practice-in-clinical-audit.

10. Hogg, P. and Cresswell, J. Interprofessional research teams in radiography – where the magic happens. *Radiography* 2021;**27**(1):S9–S13.

11. NIHR. UK Clinical Academic Training for Nurses, Midwives, AHPs and Other Health and Care Professionals: Principles and Obligations. 2021. Available at www.nihr.ac.uk/documents/uk-clinical-academic-training-for-nurses-midwives-ahps-and-other-health-and-care-professionals-principles-and-obligations/27109.

12. World Medical Association. World Medical Association Declaration of Helsinki: ethical principles for medical research involving human subjects. *JAMA* 2013;**310**(20):2191–2194.

13. NHS Health Research Authority. Research Ethics Service and Research Ethics Committees. Available at www.hra.nhs.uk/about-us/committees-and-services/res-and-recs/.

14. Gov.uk. Getting Informed Consent for User Research. Available at www.gov.uk/service-manual/user-research/getting-users-consent-for-research.

SECTION 4
SAFETY IN HEALTHCARE PROVISION

13. DEVELOPING A SAFETY CULTURE

Philip Webster

INTRODUCTION

Radiographers and technologists, as part of their training and everyday practice, undertake safety-orientated activities. This awareness makes them skilled at recognising safety improvements and adept at creating an integrated approach to safety, embedded in everyday thinking and practice. Recently, the term '**safety culture**' has been increasingly used to recognise that ongoing safety is a fundamental and dynamic process, and not just a series of actions in isolation. This approach is recognised by international agencies, government organisations and professional bodies, including the International Atomic Energy Agency (IAEA),[1] the International Society of Radiographers and Radiological Technologists (ISRRT)[2] and NHS England,[3] which produce associated publications on everyday clinical practice. These publications provide the mechanisms to embed the concept of creating, maintaining and evolving a safe environment for patients, staff and visitors to Medical Imaging and Radiotherapy Departments.

There is the ongoing need to provide an environment in which, and continuous assurance that, safety is at the forefront of the thinking and approach to care. This can be achieved through an organisational culture that assesses and seeks to improve its radiation safety. Safety is part of everyday practice and thinking and is enhanced by the creation of a **safety culture approach**, whereby individuals and the organisation consider safety in all aspects of work, and that it is an evolving process.

DOI: 9781003380078-13

Considering the elements that make a dynamic safety culture, and implementing them, provides a structure to create and develop a safe environment for patients, staff, technical support teams including medical physics staff, equipment engineers and other visitors. Medical Imaging and Radiotherapy Departments will have specific risks and safety measures that are in addition to the wider safety processes, all of which are part of the system of providing comprehensive care, for example medicines management, safeguarding, organisation-wide health and safety and staff health and wellbeing. This chapter identifies some of the common factors in creating a radiation safety culture, adapted from the IAEA safety culture traits,[1] and how they can be applied to radiation safety in Medical Imaging and Radiotherapy Departments.

CREATING A SAFETY CULTURE

A safety culture approach with an emphasis on **radiation safety** is the basis of the ongoing development of safe clinical practice in Medical Imaging and Radiotherapy Departments. This can be achieved through a combination of learning, considering real-time experience, acquired clinical practice skills, an understanding of radiation safety and implementing safety processes in clinical practice. In a strong safety culture environment, processes and procedures are considered, and they help to reduce radiation exposure. This is used in both the development and the ongoing refinement of the **International Basic Safety Standards (BSS) for Radiation Protection**,[4] in which justification, optimisation of imaging systems and dose constraints are considered. The benefits of a strong safety culture approach include lower error rates, thereby enhancing diagnostic outcomes, and the continuing aim of a reduction in exposure to radiographers, technologists and all members of the medical imaging and radiotherapy teams. The combined effect will help to improve a patient's experience and lead to an increase in efficiency across a patient's journey. Establishing a safety culture is about *a change in how we view and seek to continuously enhance processes, procedures and outcomes*. It is not just a set of rules. The objective is to dynamically support change in how we work and to improve and advance our clinical practice.

Figure 13.1 illustrates 12 factors that can contribute to creating a safety culture. In writing this chapter, with the impact of the global COVID-19 pandemic still affecting healthcare provision, the IAEA cultural traits model has been expanded to include ongoing considerations for planning in terms of workforce and disruption to the supply chain. These can have a significant impact on safety and these additional factors are applicable as part of creating an organisation resilient to a pandemic.

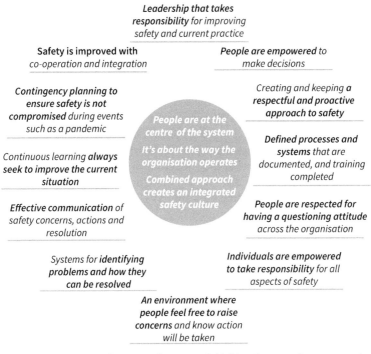

Twelve steps that can create safety culture – a continuous cycle of recognition and improvement

Leadership that takes responsibility for improving safety and current practice

Safety is improved with co-operation and integration

People are empowered to make decisions

Contingency planning to ensure safety is not compromised during events such as a pandemic

Creating and keeping **a respectful and proactive approach to safety**

People are at the centre of the system

It's about the way the organisation operates

Combined approach creates an integrated safety culture

Defined processes and systems that are documented, and training completed

Continuous learning **always seek to improve the current situation**

Effective communication of safety concerns, actions and resolution

People are respected for having a questioning attitude across the organisation

Systems for **identifying problems and how they can be resolved**

Individuals are empowered to take responsibility for all aspects of safety

An environment where people feel free to raise concerns and know action will be taken

Figure 13.1 Diagram of common factors and thinking that contribute to creating a departmental safety culture.

1. *Individuals and the organisation have a willingness to, and demonstrate, taking responsibility.* All individuals in the organisation must demonstrate taking personal and professional responsibility in considering safety issues and making changes when needed. The responsibility and authority for safety are defined in the UK Health and Safety at Work etc. Act 1974;[5] both employers and employees have a responsibility for safety. This can be achieved by identification of designated roles such as the health and safety (H&S) representative in Medical Imaging and Radiotherapy Departments, and development of documented processes including operating procedures (OPs) for equipment, sometimes referred to as standard operating procedures (SOPs), and safety data information for chemicals that may be hazardous to health.[6] These steps should include reporting relationships and team responsibilities designed to embrace and reinforce the importance of safety.

2. *Recognising safety issues and challenging poor practice.* In a safety-orientated approach, the organisation has a culture in which 'openness' is encouraged, demonstrated and present across all areas. This is found where both employees and users of the services are supported by the senior leadership team to consider current practices, raise concerns and challenge the status quo when suboptimal practices or procedures are identified. Harnessing the views of users at the service level is a powerful real-world view of what may be wrong or where improvements can be made; this is discussed in more detail in Chapter 11. This is all part of the multifaceted approach to developing and creating a dynamic safety culture approach. In the UK, this approach is explicit in the Health and Safety at Work etc. Act 1974,[5] which empowers individuals to take responsibility for, and support all actions to improve, safety.

3. *Safety-orientated decisions are part of everyday practice.* Departments should have a local safety policy that is part of the wider organisation governance process. The local guidance sets the objectives for safety procedures and identifies links with other departments and specialists in providing an integrated approach

to safety matters. The policy should be reviewed within a defined period (e.g. annually) and updated prior to the review date for any significant changes in working practice or equipment. The contribution of the team in creating and updating the policy provides invaluable insight and knowledge across the different specialisms and modalities making up a modern imaging and therapy practice.

4. *Everybody recognises the need to improve safety and it is regarded as an ongoing learning process.* The process of review and ongoing development is a key part of how an organisation operates and develops. It is a common principle in many dynamic organisations and fits well with evolving healthcare provision. It is demonstrated by a consistent approach, and it recognises opportunities to change and enhance practices to increase the overall safety. This ongoing cycle of continuous learning should be both organisational and sector-wide. The experiences of the individual and team must be recognised and actively sought for this to be effective. The organisation must provide a welcoming and supported approached to training and self-assessment, and provide processes for recognising current performance and opportunities for enhancement. The quest for improved safety must be part of the fabric of the organisation.

5. *Creating and maintaining a workplace where everybody is respected for their knowledge and experience, and as individuals.* An organisation has a key part in recognising the role of individuals in enhancing the approach to safety. This valued and respected approach is a key part of developing an organisation that is open to different views and where all perspectives are welcome. This process will be enhanced by an effective approach to communication and, when necessary, resolving issues quickly, with feedback provided as soon as possible.

6. *Making and maintaining an open environment where you can raise concerns.* There should be mechanisms across the organisation such that people feel free to raise concerns; these should be easily accessible and allow feedback to be provided to the individual raising the concern. A formalised process should provide

updates on receipt, discussion and action. Regarding resolution or improvements to the safety regime, these should be reviewed to consider the effectiveness of the intervention or change. The process for raising concerns should be tailored to the organisation and could include such initiatives as service reviews, user forums, suggestion boxes or dedicated email addresses. Depending on the organisational approach, this may include issuing anonymised reports. Additional independent mechanisms may exist, such as the local 'freedom to speak up' guardian, discussed in Chapter 6, which provides a fully independent process in the UK for reporting concerns relating to healthcare organisations.

7. *Identifying problems and solutions is part of everyday practice.* Departments and services should use a common, structured method to plan and organise activities to enable a safety-orientated approach. For each step on the patient's journey, there should be a set process to review risks and safety actions. This could include planning the workflow, examinations and safety checks prior to examinations, through to completion of the imaging or treatment and completion of the clinical record. This cycle of critical review of the full and completed action should be linked to coexisting formal requirements such as the implementation of safety checks and the critical examination of equipment as part of the UK Health and Safety Executive Ionising Radiations Regulations (IRR) 2017 Approved Code of Practice (ACOP)[7] and Ionising Radiations Regulations (Northern Ireland) (IRR [NI]) 2017.[8]

8. *Safety is always considered in developing and reviewing processes and procedures.* Consideration of safety is a requirement of all documented procedures to ensure that aspects of safety are appropriately included. This will also help to identify the equipment and resource requirements to form, for example, part of a procurement cycle for items such as personal protective equipment (PPE) or the planned preventative maintenance (PPM) programme, which ensures that equipment is properly maintained and used correctly and safely. It also includes facilities such as fire safety systems, including fire safety equipment testing.

The structured approach should include all aspects of the process: initial planning, process and control development, implementation of the process and ongoing review. Implementing a common approach and providing a detailed assessment of the safety actions, developments and enhancements can contribute to the organisational approach and enable an organisation-wide overview of safety and of the effectiveness of local actions.

9. *Safety issues and developments are known and understood.* Identification of designated roles, such as the H&S representative, should help to develop specific processes to ensure that all staff have access to information on safety issues, for example by raising awareness, providing updates on actions and delivering feedback on the resolution of issues. This may be specified by the organisation, or it may need to be developed with the department. If there is an organisation-wide process, it should be used to note any specific safety concerns that need to be escalated to the national reporting processes. In the NHS, this is the National Patient Safety Alerts (NPSA) system.[9] The outcomes and actions of a safety review or intervention should be implemented consistently using tools such as templates for documentation of OPs.

10. *Contingency planning needs to be an ongoing process.* This is to ensure continuity of services and that safety is not compromised. Major changes in the demand for care or unexpected shortages of staff and materials may affect working practices. Refer to Chapter 17 for further details on business continuity planning.

11. *Integration with other services and systems.* Safety planning, notifications, actions and structured processes are enhanced when there is integration across individual departments and organisations. This ensures that departments do not operate in isolation.

12. *Safety is a key responsibility of leadership.* Safety should be recognised by leaders at all levels. Where formal safety systems are implemented, such as H&S representatives, the duties should be formally documented and protected time should be given to carry out these duties. In all departmental policies, protocols and procedures, the recognition that safety is a key issue, together with the approach to safety management, should be stated.

THE SAFETY INFRASTRUCTURE

Healthcare organisations, and individual departments within them, will have an established overarching health and safety infrastructure. This will have been developed to provide a system of technical advice, assessment and reporting of issues and actions. Additionally, those departments delivering clinical services, such as Microbiology involvement in providing infection prevention and control (IPC) or Pharmacy involvement in providing medicines management, will have organisation-wide, as well as departmental-specific, guidance and processes to be implemented. **Figure 13.2** illustrates some of the local support and services making up the safety infrastructure within a Medical Imaging or Radiotherapy service. The safety focus specific to all Medical Imaging and Radiotherapy Departments in the UK is principally radiation safety for all modalities, magnetic resonance imaging (MRI) safety and safety when using lasers.

Radiation Safety

The key radiation safety regulatory guidance is as follows.

- ***IRR 2017 and IRR (NI) 2017.*** The legislation states the requirements relating to radiation exposure for workers and members of the public. The exposure should be restricted as far as is reasonably achievable. This is to be made possible by adopting formal legal duties, which are placed on the employing organisation, to protect its employees, and on other individuals using ionising radiation as part of their employment. This may be through working with one or more types of ionising radiation or radioactive substances. The guidance requires specific activities and duties of the employee to maintain safety. The specific requirements for both employers and employees are contained in the IRR 2017 ACOP and IRR(NI) 2017.
- ***The Ionising Radiation (Medical Exposure) Regulations 2017 (IRMER).***[10] The regulations identify several procedures and processes to provide a safety framework for individuals who

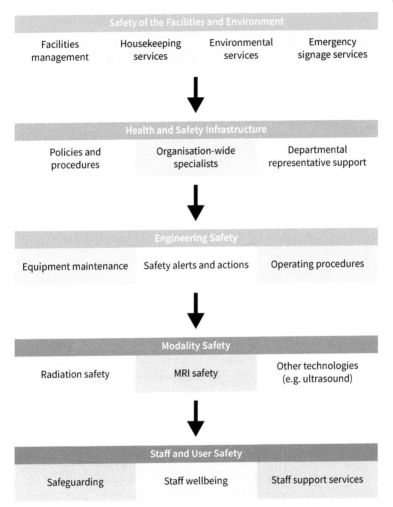

Figure 13.2 An example of some of the safety processes and support for Medical Imaging and Radiotherapy Departments.

would be exposed to ionising radiation as part of their care. This includes diagnostic imaging, radiotherapeutic procedures or for the purposes of a research study.

There are numerous specialist roles and duties within the regulations.

■ *Radiation protection advisor (RPA).* The RPA is appointed by the employing organisation to provide specialist advice in all areas of radiation protection. This includes compliance with IRR 2017, IRR (NI) 2017 and IRMER. The RPA's duties include the following.

   ○ The assessment of new equipment for radiation safety. This is called the critical examination and provides a structured assessment of the operation safety mechanisms and controls of the equipment used for diagnostic or therapeutic examinations that use ionising radiation.
   ○ Advising on practices for safe operational working through the creation of local rules.
   ○ Assessment of dose and equipment operation protocols to provide examinations in compliance with the nationally defined constraints through the application of dose reference levels (DRLs).
   ○ Advice on the design of new installations or upgrading of existing equipment in respect of radiation protection measures. This may include the radiation protection provided by the fabric of the building.
   ○ Advice on the use and application of radiation protection devices for both patient and operator.
   ○ Investigations, including dose assessment, for accidental exposure or identified increases in personnel dose.
   ○ Advice on the equipment and procedures for environmental monitoring.
   ○ Advice on the handling and use of sealed and unsealed sources used in nuclear medicine, molecular imaging and radiotherapy. Most sources for medical use are categorised as 4 (which may be used in low-dose brachytherapy) or 5 (such as the reference sources to calibrate positron emission tomography units).[11]

- *Medical physics expert (MPE).* The MPE is defined under IRMER as a formal post to provide expertise and advice for the commissioning, testing, operation and maintenance of radiation-producing equipment, including optimisation of medical exposures. This is termed 'optimisation' and is the balancing of image quality with radiation dose required to obtain a diagnostic image or therapeutic dose. Through these measures, the equipment and operational procedures provide a system to utilise the lowest dose possible to provide a diagnostic examination or radiotherapeutic exposure.
- *Radioactive waste advisor (RWA).* The RWA role is a legally defined post required for compliance with the IRR 2017. The postholder is appointed by the employing organisation as the specialist to advise on radiation protection relating to the storage and disposal of radioactive material. Appointees to the post are required to have expert knowledge and experience. The postholder provides the following services.

    o Advice on the assessment of radioactivity from distinct types of medical sources, isotopes and tracers used in providing diagnostic and radiotherapeutic services.
    o Assessment of the level of radiation, and associated radiation protection issues, in handling waste material. This must be within the specified values of the Environment Agency's permitted level of discharge or disposal of radioactive material specified in the organisational permit.

- *Radiation protection supervisor (RPS).* The RPS is appointed by the employer; the role is commonly undertaken by a radiographer or technologist after appropriate training. The duties of the role involve supervising the arrangements set out in the local rules and could include the following:

    o maintaining safe work practices, through supervision of the practices and procedures stated in the local rules;
    o ensuring that equipment is operated in accordance with the processes and guidance stated in local rules;
    o ensuring that the quality assurance (QA)/quality control (QC) regime is implemented and maintained;

- ○ maintaining formal dialogue with the appointed RPA to ensure that all relevant information on the performance or modification of imaging practices are reflected in the local rules;
- ○ ensuring personal dosimeters are available and utilised in the stated guidance;
- ○ ensuring that environmental monitoring devices are in working order and calibrated;
- ○ reporting incidents and seeking advice and guidance for immediate actions from the RPA;
- ○ supporting the RPA and clinical governance teams in the investigation of incidents.

Magnetic Resonance Imaging Safety

Guidance for the safety of MRI clinical services in the UK is published by the Medicines & Healthcare products Regulatory Agency (MHRA).[12] The specialist technical roles identified for the establishment and operation of MRI Units in the guidance are as follows:

- ■ *Magnetic resonance (MR) responsible person(s):* Responsible for operational MR safety including the provision of adequate written safety procedures, operating instructions and emergency procedures.
- ■ *MR safety officer(s):* The lead radiographer/MR technologist responsible for day-to-day implementation of MR safety policies and procedures.
- ■ *MR safety expert:* To provide advice on scientific, engineering and MR safety, to include procurement and installation advice, operating and safety procedures, QA and audit.
- ■ *MR operator:* Appropriately trained personnel for the safe operation of the MRI system.

Laser Safety

The UK Health Security Agency provides guidance on the safe use of lasers that may be used in Imaging Departments.[13] The guidance identifies the appointment of the following personnel.

- **_Laser protection advisor (LPA):_** The person with an appropriate scientific background and knowledge of laser safety. The duties of the LPA include the following:

    - maintaining a record of all class 3 and class 4 lasers, their intended use and location in the facility;
    - production of prior risk assessments for all lasers;
    - approval of the tasks and duties of the laser protection supervisors and maintaining a record of current appointees;
    - being responsible for the creation of local rules;
    - undertaking an annual inspection of areas where lasers are used and producing a written report, including the schedule of maintenance and nature of the use;
    - providing specifications and advice on equipment at the procurement stage;
    - reviewing the equipment against specification on purchase.

- **_Laser protection supervisor (LPS):_** The role of the LPS includes the following:

    - development of local rules, with the LPA, for each laser and each location in which class 3 or class 4 lasers are used;
    - ensuring that all staff involved in the use of lasers have read the local rules and collating a signed acknowledgment that they have read and will comply with them;
    - reviewing the local rules annually or when there is a change in equipment or working practices;
    - attending an approved LPS course and regular update courses as required by the LPA;
    - informing the LPA of any unsafe working practices or any changes in working practice;
    - informing the LPA of any incident or serious incident relating to the use of the laser;
    - arranging QA checks of lasers by the Medical Physics Department.

Some other devices and technologies in Medical Imaging and Radiotherapy Departments have significant safety elements, with potential hazards to both the patient and the operator. These include

ablative technology therapies such as radiofrequency nerve ablation for pain management, intraluminal microwave ablation of tissue and cryoablation. Clear operating guidance should be available to all operators and imaging staff in locations where these procedures are undertaken. This may include local rules for use and protection, OPs and QA measures.

CHAPTER SUMMARY

- Part of developing a safety culture approach is recognising that ongoing safety is a fundamental and dynamic process, and not just a series of actions in isolation.
- A safety culture for radiation safety will support a reduction in radiation dose to both staff and patients.
- The Basic Safety Standards for Radiation Protection consider justification, optimisation and dose constraints.
- There are 12 steps that create a safety culture.
- Radiation safety is regulated by key documents.
- Numerous roles are set out in the radiation regulations, all aimed at ensuring that staff and patients do not receive too much radiation exposure.
- MRI safety specialist roles ensure safe use of equipment.
- Laser safety roles ensure safe use of lasers.

REFERENCES

1. IAEA. Radiation Safety Culture Trait Talks: Handbook. Available at www.iaea.org/sites/default/files/21/01/radiation-safety-culture-trait-talks.pdf.
2. ISRRT. ISRRT Safety Culture and General Safety Guide. 2021. Available at www.isrrt.org/proffesional-practice/safety-and-safety-culture/isrrt-safety-culture-and-general-safety-guide/.
3. NHS England. Safety Culture. Available at www.england.nhs.uk/patient-safety/safety-culture/.

4. IAEA. Radiation Protection and Safety of Radiation Sources: International Basic Safety Standards. Safety Standards Series. 2014. Available at www.iaea.org/publications/8930/radiation-protection-and-safety-of-radiation-sources-international-basic-safety-standards.
5. Health and Safety at Work etc. Act 1974. Available at www.legislation.gov.uk/ukpga/1974/37/enacted.
6. Health and Safety Executive. Control of Substances Hazardous to Health (COSHH). Available at www.hse.gov.uk/coshh/.
7. Health and Safety Executive. Working with Ionising Radiation. Ionising Radiations Regulations 2017. Approved Code of Practice and Guidance. 2018. Available at www.hse.gov.uk/pubns/books/l121.htm.
8. Health and Safety Executive for Northern Ireland. Ionising Radiations Regulations (Northern Ireland) 2017 – Guidance for Notifications, Registrations and Consents. Available at www.hseni.gov.uk/sites/hseni.gov.uk/files/ionising-radiations-regulations-ni-guidance-for-notifications-registrations-and-consents.pdf.
9. NHS England. Introducing National Patient Safety Alerts. 2019. Available at www.england.nhs.uk/patient-safety/national-patient-safety-alerting-committee/.
10. Gov.uk. Ionising Radiation (Medical Exposure) Regulations 2017: Guidance. 2018. Available at www.gov.uk/government/publications/ionising-radiation-medical-exposure-regulations-2017-guidance.
11. IAEA. Sealed Radioactive Sources. 2013. Available at www.iaea.org/sites/default/files/sealedradsource1013.pdf.
12. MHRA. Safety Guidelines for Magnetic Resonance Imaging Equipment in Clinical Use. 2021. Available at https://assets.publishing.service.gov.uk/government/uploads/system/uploads/attachment_data/file/958486/MRI_guidance_2021-4-03c.pdf.
13. Gov.uk. Laser Radiation: Safety Advice. 2017. Available at www.gov.uk/government/publications/laser-radiation-safety-advice/laser-radiation-safety-advice.

14. MANAGING THE ENVIRONMENT

Philip Webster

INTRODUCTION

This chapter identifies several processes that are implemented to create a safe environment for patients, staff and visitors in the Medical Imaging and Radiotherapy Departments. It covers a wide spectrum of potential harm, including infection prevention and control (IPC), radiation dose monitoring and the many aspects of operating and managing facilities (buildings and services) to ensure that no harm comes to patients or staff. These services and specialist activities are often provided through external people or departments, such as facilities management and the infection control teams. Using IPC as an example, **Figure 14.1** illustrates the relationship between national guidance and the development of local policy and procedures.

INFECTION PREVENTION AND CONTROL

The following is an overview of the context for an IPC plan and the constituent elements of an organisational policy. During the COVID-19 pandemic, most, if not all, organisations implemented specific IPC procedures tailored to the local circumstances; reference should be

DOI: 9781003380078-14

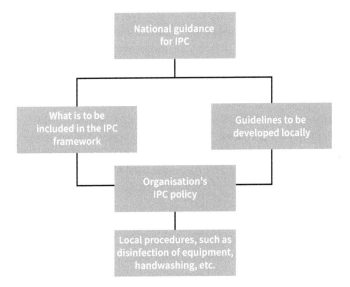

Figure 14.1 How national IPC guidance is translated into local procedures.

made to local policies and procedures. The following common terms are used:

- **IPC:** Activities, including operational, clinical and educational, to protect patients, staff and visitors from infections;
- **Healthcare-associated infection (HCAI):** An infection that is acquired because of a healthcare intervention.

The structure and guidelines for a common approach to infection control across the NHS are available in the following publications.

1. **The Health and Social Care Act 2008: Code of Practice on the Prevention and Control of Infections.**[1] This document identifies the actions all healthcare organisations should take. Those applicable to Medical Imaging and Radiotherapy Departments include the implementation of:

   a) systems to manage and monitor the prevention and control of infection;

   b) systems to provide and maintain a clean and appropriate environment to support the prevention and control of infections;

c) systems to ensure that all care workers (including contractors and volunteers) are aware of and discharge their responsibilities in the process of preventing and controlling infection;

d) systems or processes to manage staff health and wellbeing, and organisational obligation to manage infection, prevention and control.

2. ***NHS National Infection Prevention and Control Manual (NIPCM) for England.***[2] This guidance states that each healthcare organisation must implement common governance procedures that form the basis of an organisation's IPC policy. The procedures should include details of the following:

a) The arrangements for the implementation and provision of a comprehensive IPC service, usually led by an IPC team.

b) Management roles and responsibilities.

c) Infection control operational procedures, protocols and supporting guidelines. These will include the areas outlined in section one of the NIPCM:

- patient placement/assessment of infection risk;
- hand hygiene;
- respiratory and cough hygiene;
- personal protective equipment (PPE);
- safe management of the areas used to provide care, such as the imaging room or radiotherapy suite;
- safe management of equipment used in providing care;
- safe management of healthcare linen;
- safe management of blood and body fluids;
- safe disposal of waste (including sharps);
- occupational safety/managing prevention of exposure (including sharps).

The following are the key components of IPC operational procedures that are most commonly applicable to medical imaging and radiotherapy practice.

- ***Hand hygiene.*** The identification of specific hand hygiene protocols, such as the World Health Organization 10-step handwashing process.[3]

- **PPE.** Guidelines for the appropriate use of PPE, including gloves, masks, gowns and eye protection, that specify when and how to use these based on the nature of the task and potential exposure to infectious agents.
- **Isolation precautions.** Procedures for isolation and precautions appropriate to the type of infection for both staff and patients.
- **Cleaning and decontamination.** Information on types of cleaning and frequency, including methods for cleaning and disinfecting surfaces, clinical areas, medical equipment and communal areas. All equipment used in the clinical areas must be used and cleaned in accordance with the manufacturer's guidelines. Single-use equipment must be disposed of safely in accordance with the organisation's procedures and using the stated disposal containers.
- **Safe injection practices.** Including guidelines for safe injection practices, and disposal of needles and syringes.
- **Safe handling of waste.** Procedures for the segregation, handling and disposal of distinct types of waste.
- **Training and education.** Processes for training and educating staff to be fully aware of IPC procedures, including identifying the communication process for disseminating information related to infection control.

RADIATION DOSE MONITORING

There are numerous requirements for monitoring radiation dose, including radiation that exists in the environment in and around imaging rooms, that received by patients as part of their medical procedure and that received by staff when carrying out their duties. All imaging rooms using ionising radiation are classified as **controlled areas**. Entry is restricted and access given under defined working procedures, as stated in the **local rules**, which also describe the processes for use of PPE and equipment testing, for example.

Environmental Radiation Dose Monitoring

Dose monitoring is part of an organisational radiation protection strategy, undertaken as a joint approach between the Medical Imaging and

Radiotherapy Departments and the Medical Physics Department. It includes:

- environmental monitoring;
- monitoring of patient dose;
- working practice surveys;
- measurement of the radiation output of the imaging or radiotherapy equipment;
- monitoring and review of staff doses, identifying the area where a member of staff was deployed should they receive a dose on their monitoring badge.

The method and procedures for environmental assessment will be determined by the radiation protection advisor, but generally involve the use of a radiation monitoring device placed in the locality and used to assess secondary or primary radiation.

Environmental monitoring includes the identification of secondary radiation because of any leakage from the X-ray tube or scattered radiation from the imaging procedure. Dosimeters are placed on the walls external to the imaging room for a defined time period and then processed to determine if they have received a dose of radiation. Assessment of dose in areas where imaging is undertaken outside the imaging department, such as in operating theatres, intensive therapy units or special care baby units, may also involve the use of dosimeters placed strategically around the unit. If a dose is identified on the dosimeters, barriers such as walls and doors must be assessed for compliance with regulations, and an engineer must attend to assess the output of the imaging machine.

Procedures must also be in place to measure the primary radiation exposure within a defined working area, such as in an imaging room, to assess the workload that can be carried out within a fixed time, such as a day, week or month. It is used to calculate and establish if the annual dose constraints set for that location are being exceeded. Such a procedure may specify the maximum number of lateral horizontal beam hip examinations that can be performed using the erect detector in an imaging room during a set period. There must be procedures in place to ensure that this number is not exceeded.

Monitoring of the working practices in the imaging room or radiotherapy suite must be in place, and this, combined with staff dose monitoring, will ensure that exposures to staff and visitors are kept as low as possible. This could include conditional access to imaging rooms, and only in accordance with prior written arrangements, and/ or access controls such as warning lights, imaging system interlocks and interlocks at the entrance to a radiotherapy bunker.

Monitoring Patient Dose

Monitoring for record-keeping of total doses received by patients may be undertaken manually, such as recording data on a radiology information system (RIS) or electronically with integration from electronic dose monitoring systems that interface with the imaging or radiotherapy equipment. This can include imaging procedure-specific assessments of skin dose during a live procedure, such as interventional cardiac procedures or a cone beam computed tomography (CT) scan as part of image-guided radiotherapy planning. By capturing and reviewing these data, operators of radiological services demonstrate the requirement of a duty of care to make sure that patients' radiation doses are captured, stored and used to create a dose history for an individual patient. Such data should be readily available in determining the justification of further imaging. The implementation of a dose monitoring process and determining and setting the dose reference levels[4] for examinations are key actions. This is achieved by an integrated approach across the professional disciplines of radiography/radiotherapy and medical physics.

Monitoring Staff Dose

A risk assessment must be carried out for all working procedures using ionising radiation. This should consider the potential radiation exposures that an employee may receive during their routine work. There should also be an assessment of potential accidental exposure. Not all staff will require dose monitoring. Information from this process can be used to determine:

- the estimated radiation doses for each role;
- the requirement for personal dose monitoring;
- if certain employees should be designated as classified persons under the Ionising Radiations Regulations 2017 (IRR).[5]

Classified personnel will require monitoring of their dose; this is determined by identifying how likely they are to exceed three-tenths of the

Table 14.1 Dose limits for each body part.

Part of the body	Annual dose limit (mSv/year)	Annual doses above which classification would be necessary (mSv/year)
Whole body	20	6
Lens of the eye	150	45
Skin	500	150
Hands, forearms, feet and ankles	500	150

set dose limits. **Table 14.1** lists the current annual dose limits stated in Schedule 3 of the IRR.[6] The dose monitoring of staff is undertaken using agreed protocols and using certified laboratories. A range of devices are available, including electronic dose meters that provide a real-time indication of the scatter dose received. The dose monitoring results, including pregnancy status of staff working with ionising radiation, should be retained in line with local policy. If a person is employed by more than one organisation, the dose record must be shared with all employers to provide a record of the total dose received. Dose records must also be shared when moving from one employer to another so that the new employer can be sure that the new staff member does not exceed their annual limit.

FACILITIES MANAGEMENT

Facilities management is the term used to cover all services required to maintain the fabric and infrastructure of buildings and to provide a safe and fit-for-purpose environment for patients, staff and visitors. The services may be provided by the organisation's estates function or a facilities management company, and will include:

- cleaning to a specification developed with the infection control services;
- laundry services;

- lighting for both internal and external spaces;
- heating, cooling and ventilation (air handling and conditioning);
- water supply, plumbing and drainage;
- electrical supply;
- piped medical gases;
- decor and fittings such as window blinds;
- flooring, including sealed vinyl surfaces in clinical areas.

In addition to managing the infrastructure, safety systems require a maintenance and quality assurance programme, including regular testing. For example:

- fire safety – detection systems, alarms, sprinklers and extinguishers;
- emergency call and alarm systems in clinical areas;
- personal alarms, and security and security camera systems;
- emergency lighting;
- warning signs and entry barriers to controlled/supervised areas;
- environmental monitors in areas such as nuclear medicine preparation laboratories.

Contact details for routine and emergency support should be displayed in all areas.

The department is a constantly changing environment with many policies, protocols and procedures in place to enhance safety, such as regular environmental assessment for the potential hazards caused by obstructions and from the risk of slips, trips and falls. In addition, emergency and contingency plans must be in place to ensure safe evacuation in the event of an emergency or abnormal situation, such as a fire or flood. The evacuation plan should be displayed in areas throughout the department, with the nearest emergency exit indicated on the plan. In conjunction with the facilities management services, contingency plans should be developed to consider events such as electrical supply failure and heating and ventilation failure. Business continuity planning is discussed in more detail in Chapter 17.

CHAPTER SUMMARY

- IPC is related to activities, including operational, clinical and educational, to protect patients, staff and visitors from infections.
- There are numerous requirements for monitoring radiation dose, including radiation that exists in the environment in and around medical imaging or radiotherapy rooms, radiation received by patients as part of medical procedures and radiation received by staff when carrying out their duties.
- Environmental monitoring involves the identification of secondary radiation outside the medical imaging or radiotherapy treatment room.
- Dose constraints will be applied to individual imaging rooms, thereby determining the number of examinations that may be performed in a set time frame.
- Patient dose monitoring for imaging is generally undertaken on an RIS or recorded in an appropriate radiotherapy system.
- Some staff may be categorised as classified personnel; they will require radiation dose monitoring and medical surveillance by an appointed doctor.
- Facilities management includes the maintenance of the fabric and infrastructure of buildings, as well as the management of safety systems.

REFERENCES

1. Gov.uk. Health and Social Care Act 2008: Code of Practice on the Prevention and Control of Infections. 2022. Available at www.gov.uk/government/publications/the-health-and-social-care-act-2008-code-of-practice-on-the-prevention-and-control-of-infections-and-related-guidance.
2. NHS England. National Infection Prevention and Control Manual (NIPCM) for England. 2024. Available at www.england.nhs.uk/national-infection-prevention-and-control-manual-nipcm-for-england.

3. World Health Organization. How to Handwash? 2009. Available at www.who.int/docs/default-source/patient-safety/how-to-handwash-poster.pdf?sfvrsn=7004a09d_2.
4. Gov.uk. National Diagnostic Reference Levels (NDRLs) from 13 October 2022. Available at www.gov.uk/government/publications/diagnostic-radiology-national-diagnostic-reference-levels-ndrls/ndrl.
5. The Ionising Radiations Regulations 2017. Available at www.legislation.gov.uk/uksi/2017/1075/contents.
6. The Ionising Radiations Regulations 2017: Schedule 3. Available at www.legislation.gov.uk/uksi/2017/1075/schedule/3/.

15. RISK AND INCIDENT MANAGEMENT

Louise Kemp

INTRODUCTION

Risk can be defined as the possibility of an event taking place, as a result of an identified hazard, that will impact on the achievement of organisational objectives, such as providing safe care to patients. Risk impact can be positive or negative, although risks are more generally identified in terms of a negative or harmful impact. It is better to identify risk before harm occurs through proactive risk assessments and preventative action. However, incidents that cause harm, or that have the potential to cause harm, do occur and the resultant investigation is likely to identify an underlying risk that needs to be managed. Consequently, risks and incidents are inextricably linked. By identifying and managing risk appropriately, the likelihood of incidents occurring is minimised; likewise, by managing any incident that does occur, a risk assessment can take place with corrective actions to prevent similar incidents.

RISK MANAGEMENT

Risk management involves identifying potential hazards before they occur and putting measures in place to prevent them from occurring and/or to minimise the impact if they do. It is a way of providing

DOI: 9781003380078-15

assurance – an evidence-based indication of quality and safety – to the organisation by demonstrating that risks are well controlled. Effective risk management leads to improved patient/staff safety and supports business planning, decision-making and prioritisation. It is common for business cases to include details of risks mitigated as part of the justification for the case.

Risk is a function of the **likelihood** of a harm happening and the level of **impact** if it does happen. Risks may be categorised according to the business or management area affected and may fall under one of the following areas:

- clinical;
- strategic;
- financial;
- reputational;
- performance;
- operational;
- business;
- organisational;
- information security.

Risk impact will differ according to the risk type. For example, a catastrophic financial risk may be a £1M+ claim or loss, whereas a reputational risk may involve media coverage at national level or a devastating Care Quality Commission (CQC) report.

The organisational **risk management framework or strategy** will detail the responsibilities, the approach to managing risk, risk appetite and reporting and escalation (increasing the level of authority overseeing the risk according to the risk score) processes. **Risk appetite** describes the level of risk the organisation is willing to accept in order to achieve its objectives. This can vary depending on the circumstances: there may be a low risk appetite when it comes to patient safety, but a greater willingness to tolerate risk when it comes to delivering innovation or improvement. Risk appetite helps to set boundaries in terms of acceptable levels of risk and informs the risk management approach.

A number of steps are involved in management of risk.

1. *Identify the risk.* Risks may be identified proactively (thinking about what could happen, such as actively 'horizon scanning', i.e. using knowledge of future developments and trends to look for potential risks, or risk assessing a new procedure or project) or reactively (reflecting and learning from something that has happened, such as an incident or complaint). An owner of the risk should be identified – somebody within the organisation with the authority to manage the risk.

2. *Assess and evaluate.* Once identified, the risk can be assessed in terms of the possible impact or harm, and the scale of the risk. The risk can be described in terms of the possible outcome(s):

   ▪ IF (*risk event*) happens THEN (*consequence/harm*) could occur.

This should be clearly articulated in terms of the effect on patients, public, staff, service and organisation. The risk score should be calculated by considering the current state, taking account of existing controls but not proposed or future controls. It is calculated by multiplying the **likelihood** of the harm materialising (**Table 15.1**) by the **impact** of the risk should it happen (**Table 15.2**), to produce an estimated level of risk. Risk scoring can be highly subjective so the use of a predefined risk matrix with clear descriptors can be useful to help quantify or qualify each score in relation to the impact of the risk. The risk score can then be calculated (**Table 15.3**). Risk scoring helps to identify priorities in terms of managing risk and where resources should be focused, ensuring actions are proportionate to the level of risk.

Risk evaluation involves deciding how best to manage the risk (including consideration of what might happen if no action were taken to treat the risk), what controls are in place already to reduce the risk, what additional controls/actions are needed and what the residual or target risk score would be if all controls were in place. This will help to determine whether the proposed controls are sufficient to manage the risk. Decisions on risk treatment will be informed by the organisational risk appetite.

Table 15.1 Example of assessment of risk likelihood.

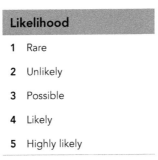

Likelihood	
1	Rare
2	Unlikely
3	Possible
4	Likely
5	Highly likely

Table 15.2 Example of a risk matrix for assessing the impact of risks associated with injury, financial position or service delivery.

	Impact				
Category	**1** **Insignificant**	**2** **Minor**	**3** **Moderate**	**4** **Major**	**5** **Catastrophic**
Injury	No injury sustained	First aid required, no lasting effects; no overnight stay	Significant but not permanent harm; medical treatment required; short-term hospital stay required	Long-term harm/ incapacity or prolonged hospital stay	Death or multiple major injuries
Finance	<£1,000 loss	£1,000– £10,000 loss	£10,000– £100,000 loss	£100,000– £1M loss	>£1M loss
Service delivery	Short-term disruption; no impact on patient care	Short-term loss of service; minor impact on patient care	Ongoing disruption; moderate impact on patient care	Ongoing disruption to service; significant impact on patient care	Long-term or permanent loss of service; severe impact on patient care

Table 15.3 Calculation of risk score and severity.

	Impact				
Likelihood	Insignificant	Minor	Moderate	Major	Catastrophic
1 Rare	1	2	2	4	5
2 Unlikely	2	4	6	8	10
3 Possible	3	6	9	12	15
4 Likely	4	8	12	16	20
5 Highly likely	5	10	15	20	25

	Low risk
	Medium risk
	Medium-high risk
	High risk

3. **Reduce the risk.** There are four ways to treat a risk:
   a) **Avoid/terminate.** Can the risk be eliminated altogether?
   b) **Reduce.** What measures can be put in place to reduce either the likelihood or the impact of the risk?
   c) **Transfer.** Can the risk be moved to another party, for example taking out insurance on equipment?
   d) **Accept/tolerate.** If a risk cannot be avoided, reduced or transferred, an organisation may choose to accept the risk, depending on the risk appetite and the risk score. If a risk score is low, treatment may not be required, and the risk may be considered acceptable to the delivery of services.

   If it is identified that a risk requires further action to reduce the likelihood and/or impact, an action plan should be put in place. The actions must have an identified owner and should be specific, measurable, achievable, relevant and time-bound (SMART).

4. **Monitor and review.** Once the approach to managing a risk has been established, it will need to be monitored for progress and effectiveness. The frequency of review will be dependent on the

risk score, with higher-scoring risks (such as those ≥15) requiring more regular oversight, maybe fortnightly or monthly, whereas a very low-scoring risk (perhaps ≤3) may only need reviewing annually (see Table 15.3). When reviewing a risk, consider the following:

- Is the risk still valid – does the risk still exist?
- Has the likelihood or impact changed?
- Is there change of ownership?
- Are mitigating actions on track? Do target dates need to be amended or actions followed up?
- Details of current position/progress/any changes made to the risk?
- Have the controls and actions been completed; can the risk be closed?

5. *Reporting and escalation*. When a risk is identified, it should be added to a risk register. This ensures that there is regular oversight of all risks. High-scoring risks should be regularly monitored as part of the departmental quality and governance approach. They may be flagged to divisional and/or corporate teams and may also be added to divisional or corporate-level risk registers. The organisational risk policy or framework will define what a high-scoring risk is and at what risk forums they will be reviewed, such as local departmental level, directorate level or organisational level.

6. *Closure.* A risk may be closed when it has been successfully treated, avoided, transferred or accepted. The circumstances around risk closure should be documented formally on the risk register as part of the audit trail to show the complete management of the risk.

The Risk Register

A risk register is a working document (or system) that supports the management of risks. The risk register aids decision-making and planning by highlighting risk priorities. The organisation may have different types of risk registers in place, for example:

- *Departmental:* operational service risks;

- **Directorate/divisional:** risks to achieving local divisional business or strategic objectives;
- **Corporate:** risks to delivery of core business and achievement of corporate objectives.

The risk register will usually capture the following, at a minimum:

- **Date:** the date that the risk was identified and added to the register;
- **Title** and **description** of the risk: describe what could happen if the risk materialised, using the 'IF (*risk event*) happens THEN (*consequence/harm*) could occur' means of outlining this;
- **Likelihood:** a measure of how likely the risk is to materialise;
- **Impact:** a measure of the level of impact if the risk does materialise;
- **Risk rating/score:** calculated by using the likelihood score multiplied by the impact score of the risk;
- **Risk owner:** the individual responsible for managing and controlling the risk (although not necessarily for carrying out the mitigating actions);
- **Controls:** it is necessary to outline the measures in place to reduce the risk in terms of likelihood, impact or both;
- **Action plan:** identify further controls and actions needed to reduce or remove the risk, including the action owner(s) and the timescales for completion;
- **Residual** or **target score:** this is the expected risk score once all controls/mitigating actions have been implemented and the risk cannot be reduced any further.

Risk registers are dynamic documents and should undergo regular review in line with the organisational risk management policy. Different risks may be reviewed at different times and in different forums, as outlined above. They may also be reviewed and updated more frequently than the defined review periods when circumstances change, affecting the level of oversight required. The risk owner is usually responsible for ensuring review of individual risks.

An Example Risk Assessment

Take the scenario of a hole in the roof of the department causing water to enter when it rains. The risk is NOT that there is a hole in the roof.

The risk is: *IF* rainwater comes in through the hole in the roof, *THEN* it might cause staff or patients to slip and be injured. The LIKELIHOOD being assessed is not of the roof leaking, but of someone slipping and being injured as a result, although various factors would need to be considered.

- *Location:* if this is in a busy corridor used by staff and patients, the likelihood of slipping and injury is higher than if the hole is in the corner of a staff room with limited traffic.
- *Frequency/scale:* is there a large puddle every time it rains or does the leak occur only in very severe weather? If the leak is infrequent, the likelihood of someone slipping in a puddle is reduced.

In this case, the hole is above the entrance to the department, causing a pool of water to collect in the middle of the corridor each time there is minor rain. The LIKELIHOOD of someone slipping could be classed as POSSIBLE (score of 3). When determining IMPACT, the person assessing the risk should consider what *could* happen – a 'worst-case scenario' – rather than what is most likely to happen: in this example it might be that someone *could* break a bone by falling, leading to, at best, immobilisation and, at worst, surgical treatment. If we refer to the risk matrix for injuries (**Table 15.4**), a broken bone needing surgical intervention could reasonably be scored as a 3. The overall score for this risk would be:

$$\text{LIKELIHOOD} \times \text{IMPACT} = 3 \times 3 = 9$$

According to the risk-scoring matrix (see Table 15.3), this would be described as a medium-high risk.

Sometimes more than one category might apply; for example, the slip injury may also result in a complaint or litigation. The impact used should be that of the highest-scoring category descriptor defined in the risk matrix.

Existing controls to reduce the risk of injury might be use of warning signs, barriers or diversions. **Table 15.5** outlines a possible long-term action plan for this risk.

Once the action plan has been implemented, the risk can be reassessed and rescored. The action plan has now become a control. Once the hole has been repaired, the risk is no longer applicable; the risk has been managed and can be closed on the risk register.

Table 15.4 Risk matrix example for injuries.

Score	Impact
1	No injury sustained
2	Minor injury: first aid required, no lasting effects; no overnight stay
3	Moderate injury: significant but not permanent harm; medical treatment required; short-term hospital stay required
4	Major injury: long-term harm/incapacity; prolonged hospital stay
5	Death or multiple major injuries

Table 15.5 Example of a long-term action plan for the scenario.

Control	Actions	Owner	Timescale
Temporary fix of the hole in the roof	Contact estates to put urgent temporary covering in place while permanent fix is organised	AB	3 days
Fix the hole in the roof	Contact estates team for a quote for the work to be carried out	AB	4 weeks
Fix the hole in the roof	Raise a job with estates once the quote for the work has been approved	CD	8 weeks

INCIDENT MANAGEMENT

An incident is an unintended or unexpected event (including an omission) in healthcare that caused harm, or had the potential to cause harm, to one or more patients. Harm can be defined as a negative or adverse effect that happens as a direct result of care or treatment provided, or by the failure to provide care or treatment. Harm may be physical or psychological. Degrees of harm are defined by the NHSE[1] as follows:

- **No harm:** the incident had the potential to cause harm, but was prevented (near miss) OR incident took place but no harm occurred;

- *Low:* minimal harm; minor treatment required;
- *Moderate:* significant (but not permanent) harm; further treatment required;
- *Severe:* permanent harm;
- *Death:* the incident directly resulted in the death of the patient(s).

Some incidents may be classed as **never events**. This is an incident that causes (or has the potential to cause) serious harm or death to a patient where an existing guideline has not been followed, for example wrong-site surgery or positioning of a nasogastric tube in the respiratory tract followed by administration of feed. Never events are preventable because national guidance or safety recommendations are already available and should have been adopted by the organisation. Never events must undergo patient safety incident investigation (PSII).

In the event of any incident occurring, the following should take place:

- take immediate action to ensure safety of patients, staff and public;
- report the incident as soon as possible via the organisational incident reporting system in line with the organisation's incident reporting policy;
- provide support to those involved if needed;
- investigate what happened and why it happened;
- put in place a sustainable improvement plan;
- share learning with others.

Incident Reporting

Incident reporting helps organisations to improve quality and safety by learning from mistakes and putting measures in place to prevent recurrence. Reporting incidents is not an indication of an unsafe environment; it is a positive indication of a safety culture. In fact, lack of incident reporting may serve as a warning flag that learning and improvement are not taking place. Incident management forms part of the CQC key lines of enquiry (KLOE), a framework of standards used to evaluate the quality of care in organisations.[2] Most organisations will have an incident reporting system in place. When recording an incident, it is usual to capture the following:

- date and time the incident occurred;

- person(s) involved;
- location of incident – the location where the incident was identified may be different to the location where it took place or originated;
- type of incident/incident categorisation;
- description of the incident;
- immediate action taken;
- initial assessment of level of impact/harm;
- whether duty of candour is required.

Incident Investigation

Once identified, an incident should be investigated so that actions can be put in place to make sure systems or environments are safe, to reduce risks to others if the incident recurs and to prevent the incident recurring. It should be noted that a near-miss incident with the potential to cause significant harm may be categorised as no harm, but could need a high priority of investigation.

Incident investigation should focus on the following.

- What happened – gathering the facts about the incident.
- How it happened – what were the steps leading up to and including the incident?
- Why it happened – looking at the factors affecting the event.
- Whether **duty of candour** is required.
- Identifying any factors that minimised, or could have minimised, harm.
- Evaluation of the actual harm caused.
- Actions and learning from the incident – what could be put in place to prevent the incident recurring or to minimise the harm caused?

The NHS no longer distinguishes between incidents and serious incidents; instead, the **Patient Safety Incident Response Framework** (PSIRF)[3] advocates 'a proportionate approach to responding to patient safety incidents by ensuring resources allocated to learning are balanced with those needed to deliver improvement'. This builds a closer relationship between quality improvement and learning from incidents and complaints, promoting the use of quality data to determine response priorities and compassionate engagement and involvement of those affected. The PSIRF requires organisations to develop a patient safety incident response policy that details the local incident response decision-making processes; the approach to improvement planning; and how staff, patients and carers will be involved in the learning.

The NHS promotes a 'systems-based' approach to PSII whereby all factors contributing towards the incident are considered, rather than simply looking for the 'root cause' or at the actions of individuals involved. The **System Engineering Initiative for Patient Safety** (SEIPS)[4] framework is the incident investigation framework endorsed by PSIRF; it seeks to understand a range of different factors within complex systems such as technology, tasks, people and environment.

Incident Learning

Learning from incidents is a key element of incident management, as it leads to changes being implemented to ensure that systems and processes are as safe as possible and to reduce the likelihood of recurrence. There should be mechanisms in place in the department and organisation to ensure timely sharing of actions, learning and changes to work practices to all staff who may need to be aware, not just to those involved or affected. The PSIRF promotes the use of the following 'learning response' methods.

- *Swarm huddle:* the staff involved come together immediately post-incident to capture information on what happened, to consider how to reduce risk and to generate learning, for example post-cardiac arrest.
- *After-action review (AAR):* focused discussion exploring what happened, what should have happened, what went well and what could be improved. This may be in response to a positive or a negative event.
- *PSII:* detailed review in response to patient safety or near-miss incidents looking at what happened and how, aimed at understanding decisions and actions that took place and to identify learning.
- *Multidisciplinary team (MDT) review:* the MDT explores in depth multiple similar patient safety incidents by looking at themes or pathways, to identify gaps and any learning needed, for example medication error.

The process of 'appreciative inquiry' aims to implement positive change and 'learning from excellence' as part of the incident response, learning through identifying areas of strength and good practice within a system, and finding ways to grow and expand these.

There are national sources of information in the UK that can contribute to learning from incidents.

■ The 'Learn From Patient Safety Events' (LFPSE) service, which has replaced the National Reporting and Learning System (NRLS) and the Strategic Executive Information System (StEIS). LFPSE records and analyses patient safety events.
■ National Patient Safety Alerts (NPSA): information from NHS England regarding safety-critical risks.
■ 'Prevention of future deaths' reports, also known as Regulation 28, are issued to organisations during or following an inquest where the coroner believes that action is needed to prevent similar deaths occurring in future. These are published on the judiciary website.[5]

The culture in an organisation shapes the values and behaviours of the people that work in it, which in turn affects the quality and safety of care delivered. Organisations with a 'just culture' understand that human errors can occur and considers how the wider system might have contributed to incidents occurring, encouraging those involved to speak up when things go wrong without being fearful of negative consequences. Instead, staff feel encouraged and supported to learn from mistakes. A just culture will also hold people to account where appropriate, such as in the case of negligent or deliberately dangerous acts.

Human Factors

Human factors, sometimes known as ergonomics, refers to things that influence the behaviours of people in the workplace, and the impact of these behaviours on safety. These may relate to:

■ the environment;
■ systems and processes;
■ staff fatigue;
■ poor equipment design;
■ interruptions.

Understanding the human factors that contribute to incidents allows us to redesign these elements to reduce the likelihood of the incident recurring. For example, there are well-documented examples whereby labelling on different medicines with very similar appearances led to the wrong medication being administered, sometimes with catastrophic implications for the patient. Changing the packaging meant that these errors were less likely to occur.

Duty of Candour

In 2013 the Francis Inquiry[6] identified 'significant failings in openness and transparency' at a trust in the UK and recommended the introduction of a statutory 'duty of candour' for healthcare providers in addition to that required of registered healthcare practitioners as part of their professional standards.[7] The UK Health and Care Professions Council (HCPC) states that radiographers have 'an ethical responsibility to be open and honest with service users and their employers when things go wrong with a person's care', known as the professional duty of candour.[8] The statutory duty of candour[7] was enacted in 2014 for NHS organisations, requiring organisations to be open and transparent with patients about their care and treatment, including informing patients as soon as possible that a 'notifiable incident' has occurred in relation to their care. A 'notifiable safety incident' is a specific term defined in the duty of candour regulation when an incident meets *all three* of the following criteria:

- was unintended or unexpected;
- occurred during the provision of a CQC-regulated activity;
- resulted in, or could have resulted in, death or severe/moderate harm.

The patient or their representative should be invited to discuss:

- what has happened regarding their care and any implications;
- what investigation(s) will take place and expected timescales.

This must be followed up in writing with a written apology and any update on the investigation. A record of all communication (including attempted communication) must be kept. The apology is not an admission of liability.

223

Freedom to Speak Up

The Francis Inquiry identified an organisational culture where staff did not feel confident in raising concerns about poor standards of care. The 2015 'Freedom to Speak Up' (FTSU) review was again chaired by Sir Robert Francis QC and made a series of recommendations around organisational culture and the handling of the raising of concerns.[9] The National Guardian's Office and FTSU guardians were established in 2016 as impartial and independent roles to support staff and volunteers to speak up without fear of reprisal, to encourage a positive culture around speaking up and to promote learning and improvement around quality and patient care as a result of speaking up. All organisations providing NHS services under the standard NHS contract must appoint a FTSU guardian.

CHAPTER SUMMARY

- Risk is the possibility of an event taking place as a result of an identified hazard.
- Proactive risk assessment and preventative action will minimise the impact of any subsequent incident.
- Risk management involves identifying and evaluating the risk before treating the risk.
- A risk register will support the management of organisational risks, and support decision-making in relation to risk priorities.
- An incident is an event that is unintended or unexpected and has the potential to, or does, cause actual harm.
- Incident management involves investigating a reported incident to understand what, why and how the incident occurred.
- A 'never event' is an incident that has the potential to, or does, cause serious harm or death where a guideline has not been followed.
- Understanding human factors that contribute to incidents enables an intervention aimed at reducing the likelihood of that incident occurring.

- The statutory duty of candour for healthcare professionals requires openness and honesty with service users when things go wrong.
- FTSU guardians are a source of impartial and independent support to enable staff to speak up freely and without fear.

FURTHER READING

- NHS England and NHS Improvement. The NHS Patient Safety Strategy: Safer Culture, Safer Systems, Safer Patients. Available at www.england.nhs.uk/wp-content/uploads/2020/08/190708_Patient_Safety_Strategy_for_website_v4.pdf.
- NHS Improvement. Never Events Policy and Framework. Available at www.england.nhs.uk/wp-content/uploads/2020/11/Revised-Never-Events-policy-and-framework-FINAL.pdf.
- NHS England. Patient Safety Incident Response Framework Supporting Guidance: Guide to Responding Proportionately to Patient Safety Incidents. Available at www.england.nhs.uk/wp-content/uploads/2022/08/B1465-3.-Guide-to-responding-proportionately-to-patient-safety-incidents-v1-FINAL.pdf.
- NHS. A Just Culture Guide. Available at www.england.nhs.uk/wp-content/uploads/2021/02/NHS_0932_JC_Poster_A3.pdf.
- NHS England. Patient Safety Incident Investigation. Version 1, August 2022. Available at www.england.nhs.uk/wp-content/uploads/2022/08/B1465-PSII-overview-v1-FINAL.pdf.

REFERENCES

1. NHS England. Policy Guidance on Recording Patient Safety Events and Levels of Harm. 2023. Available at www.england.nhs.uk/long-read/policy-guidance-on-recording-patient-safety-events-and-levels-of-harm/.
2. CQC. Key Lines of Enquiry, Prompts and Ratings Characteristics for Adult Social Care Services. Available at www.cqc.org.uk/sites/default/files/20171020_adult_social_care_kloes_prompts_and_characteristics_final.pdf.

3. NHS England. Patient Safety Incident Response Framework. Available at www.england.nhs.uk/wp-content/uploads/2022/08/B1465-1.-PSIRF-v1-FINAL.pdf.
4. NHS England. SEIPS Quick Reference Guide and Work System Explorer. Available at www.england.nhs.uk/wp-content/uploads/2022/08/B1465-SEIPS-quick-reference-and-work-system-explorer-v1-FINAL.pdf.
5. Courts and Tribunals Judiciary. Reports to Prevent Future Deaths. Available at www.judiciary.uk/courts-and-tribunals/coroners-courts/reports-to-prevent-future-deaths/.
6. Francis, R. Report of the Mid Staffordshire NHS Foundation Trust Public Inquiry: Executive Summary. Available at https://assets.publishing.service.gov.uk/government/uploads/system/uploads/attachment_data/file/279124/0947.pdf.
7. CQC. Regulation 20: Duty of Candour. Available at www.cqc.org.uk/guidance-providers/all-services/regulation-20-duty-candour.
8. HCPC. Standards of Conduct, Performance and Ethics. Available at www.hcpc-uk.org/globalassets/resources/standards/standards-of-conduct-performance-and-ethics.pdf.
9. Francis, R. Freedom to Speak Up: An Independent Review into Creating an Open and Honest Reporting Culture in the NHS. 2015. Available at http://freedomtospeakup.org.uk/wp-content/uploads/2014/07/F2SU_web.pdf.

16. INFORMATICS

Louise Kemp and Philip Webster

INTRODUCTION

Healthcare informatics is a term used to describe the use of information and technology in the acquisition, processing and analysis of patient data to deliver and improve healthcare. '**Data**' is defined as follows:

> *information, especially facts or numbers, collected to be examined and considered and used to help decision-making.*[1]

When a patient attends the Medical Imaging or Radiotherapy Department, data about them and their visit are collected. This falls into three broad categories:

- **Demographic:**
  - name;
  - address;
  - date of birth;
  - gender.
- **Administrative:**
  - examination undertaken;
  - appointments made.
- **Medical:**
  - referrals made;
  - images;
  - reports;
  - radiotherapy and treatment plans.

DOI: 9781003380078-16

Significant volumes of data are generated in healthcare, which can be used to support future developments or benchmark against other organisations. This data is managed by specialist teams with knowledge of healthcare informatics and business intelligence (BI).

This chapter identifies the types of systems and data in use in Medical Imaging and Radiotherapy Departments, including the role of artificial intelligence (AI), and how those data are managed safely. Whenever data are being used, data protection and confidentiality are essential, and processes must be in place to limit access to those who have legitimate reasons to access the data.

IMAGING AND INFORMATION SYSTEMS

Medical imaging and radiotherapy are widely recognised as highly technologically enabled specialties that use a range of digital systems and data across the full diagnostic imaging and radiotherapy pathways, from referral to treatment and results. Information systems are used to collect, store, manage and share such healthcare data. The following are those most commonly found in medical imaging and radiotherapy workflows.

- **Radiology information system (RIS).** The RIS receives/records patient referrals, handles scheduling and appointments, records information on examination history and radiation dose and provides reporting functionality, management and storage. The RIS may provide additional support for the management of imaging pathways.
- **Radiotherapy record-and-verify system (RVS).** The RVS stores information on treatment planning and delivery.
- **Picture archiving and communication system (PACS).** PACS stores images and reports, and provides image manipulation and reporting functionality.
- **Electronic patient record (EPR).** The EPR is a hospital-wide system that manages and stores patient medical records from multiple specialties. This forms the patient's master clinical record.

228

■ *Patient administration system (PAS)*. The PAS records non-clinical patient information, such as name, date of birth and their home address, and information in relation to their next of kin.

■ *Master patient index (MPI)*. The MPI manages patient identifiers (IDs) across separate administrative, financial and clinical systems. It records non-clinical data associated with clinical attendances, such as the date and length of a hospital stay. An enterprise MPI (EMPI) manages these records across regions or multiple organisations.

■ *Ordercomms/Order Communications and Results Reporting (OCRR)*. The Ordercomms or OCRR handles electronic requests/referrals and the transfer of results to referring clinicians.

■ *Artificial intelligence.* AI is gaining momentum in medical imaging and radiotherapy services. It involves the simulation of human processes by computer systems. AI can be capable of machine learning, that is using data to learn and improve, such as voice recognition software, which improves as it learns to recognise the individual user's voice and commands. Not all AI involves machine learning – many systems work by automating routine or repetitive tasks to reduce errors and increase efficiency. In imaging, AI is commonly associated with image reporting algorithms such as identification of chest pathologies, fracture detection or head computed tomography (CT) interpretation. These are relatively new technologies with the potential to increase efficiency in the reporting workflow. AI is also emerging as a tool for different applications in the radiotherapy workflow, such as automatic tumour and organ-at-risk (OAR) segmentation, or adaptive planning workflows that allow treatment to respond to changes in the patient condition.

There has been some concern that AI could eventually replace reporting by radiologists and radiographers. Although AI has proved to be similar in specificity and sensitivity to human reporters in pathology identification, it is still being validated for safety and how it should be used to maximise its benefits. Ultimately, the expertise of the reporter lies in applying their breadth of knowledge to the patient's context and pathway. It seems more likely that AI will provide solutions to improve accuracy and efficiency, thereby enhancing the reporting process, rather than replacing the radiologist or reporting radiographer. AI-generated reports may provide value through clinical decision support, particularly in an out-of-hours situation and/or where clinicians are less experienced in image review, although there is still much research to be done in this area. There are opportunities for AI across the full patient pathway, from referral to results, for example:

- automatic scheduling;
- image optimisation;
- triage for reporting priorities;
- intelligent report allocation;
- clinical decision support;
- pathology detection and tumour classification;
- report alerts and notifications.

BUSINESS INTELLIGENCE

BI is a term used to describe the use of software that can ingest large volumes of data and provide an overview and interpretation in the form of dashboards, reports and charts. These help the senior leadership team to make 'data-driven' operational and strategic decisions and support real-time monitoring of activity, identification of trends and business/financial planning. Data from imaging systems provide vital information on the patient journey, for example evidencing performance (waiting times or report turnaround) and activity (modality numbers or referral trends). Data extracted are only as accurate as data inputted. To be relevant, data should be:

- **Timely:** captured at the time of the event so that details are not forgotten or incorrectly recalled;
- **Consistent:** recorded in the same way each time to ensure comparability;
- **Accurate:** reflect the real-world event or position;
- **Valid:** stored in the correct format;
- **Complete:** all information is captured; there are no gaps in the data.

Policies and procedures must be in place to ensure a standardised approach to data entry, meaning information is both accessible and comparable. These data enable the senior leadership team to identify areas for improvement, to develop future plans for staff and equipment, to support financial and operational decisions and to accurately complete incident and complaint investigations. It also enables **benchmarking**, a process of evaluation against similar organisations, allowing comparison in terms of resources, productivity, performance, workforce metrics and other measures, with a view to identifying areas of good practice and opportunities for improvement. The **Model Health System** (MHS) is a digital service designed to support benchmarking in order to identify variation and work towards reducing inequality. MHS imaging data are derived from the annual National Imaging Data Collection, which compiles detailed information from an organisation in terms of activity, performance, capacity, equipment and workforce. Similar benchmarking information can also be derived from the **Diagnostic Imaging Dataset** (DID), a monthly collection of examination-specific data for medical imaging activity in England, and the **Radiotherapy Data Set** (RTDS), the national standard for radiotherapy data collection in the NHS. All NHS-funded providers of radiotherapy services in England are required to submit monthly data against nationally defined standards.

INFORMATION TECHNOLOGY SYSTEM SECURITY

There are strict requirements from NHS England to ensure system and data security in NHS organisations, which may be subject to fines if they do not comply. These rules are in place to ensure that patient data are not compromised, either by loss or theft, or by lack of access to systems at the point of care, for example by the system becoming infected with a virus.

All information technology (IT) equipment, including that installed on medical imaging and radiotherapy devices such as CT or X-ray equipment, should be kept up to date with software versions and security patches. This can prove challenging within equipment refresh cycles due to the complexities of manufacturer testing against each new release or where the software installed is no longer supported, but the equipment is not yet due for replacement. For this reason, medical imaging and radiotherapy equipment may be a source of vulnerability to cyberattack. In addition to preventative and security measures, processes should be in place to ensure business continuity should this happen.

Medical imaging and radiotherapy modalities use IT hardware, operating systems and specialist modality-specific software to operate, store, manipulate and share the images produced. Modality systems may be classed as medical devices, which are strictly regulated, including in terms of modifications (such as software upgrades), to ensure patient safety is maintained. This can cause challenges in managing **digital security** requirements for devices on the organisation's network, as operating system and security patches/upgrades may not form part of the modality contractual provision, and indeed can be problematic for suppliers to manage and test under the broad range of possible external environments. Remote access may also be required for equipment service management, giving rise to further network security complexities. Installation and management of equipment requires co-ordination and a mutually respectful working relationship between the IT department, the Medical Imaging or Radiotherapy Department and the equipment supplier.

PROTECTION OF INFORMATION

The protection of an individual's information as a patient, employee or member of the public is subject to laws in many countries. In the European Union (EU), the legal framework is the **General Data Protection Regulation** (GDPR).[2] This requirement is followed in UK law through the Data Protection Act 2018, which requires compliance with the regulations.[3] The GDPR regulates the way in which personal data can be handled, giving individuals more control over their personal information. It defines seven principles (**Figure 16.1**) of how data are collected, used and stored, which organisations are required to prove they comply with.

Individuals have the right to find out what information is held about them. This includes the right to:

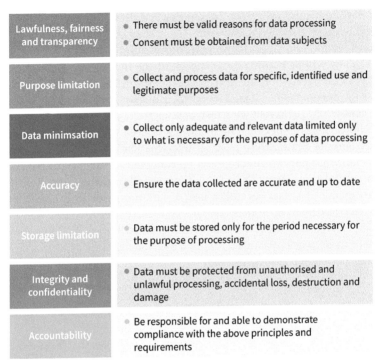

Lawfulness, fairness and transparency	• There must be valid reasons for data processing • Consent must be obtained from data subjects
Purpose limitation	• Collect and process data for specific, identified use and legitimate purposes
Data minimsation	• Collect only adequate and relevant data limited only to what is necessary for the purpose of data processing
Accuracy	• Ensure the data collected are accurate and up to date
Storage limitation	• Data must be stored only for the period necessary for the purpose of processing
Integrity and confidentiality	• Data must be protected from unauthorised and unlawful processing, accidental loss, destruction and damage
Accountability	• Be responsible for and able to demonstrate compliance with the above principles and requirements

Figure 16.1 Principles of GDPR.

- be told about how their data are being used;
- obtain access to their personal data;
- correct inaccurate information;
- have data removed;
- stop or restrict the processing of data;
- data portability (access to data);
- opt out of data processing (in certain circumstances).

The UK national data opt-out allows a patient to decide whether they want their confidential information to be used beyond individual care for research and planning.

There are two types of authority defined in the regulations based on how they collect and use personal data: data controller and data processor. This may refer to a person, public authority, agency or other body.[2]

233

A **data controller** is an organisation that has decided to collect or process personal data. They will define what data should be collected and from whom, and what the purpose or outcome of the processing will be. They will be making decisions about the individuals concerned as part of, or because of, the processing. They will appoint a data processor to process the personal data on their behalf. A **data processor** is an organisation that is following instructions from someone else regarding the processing of personal data. They are given the personal data by a customer or similar third party or told what data to collect and do not decide what personal data should be collected, or the lawful basis for the use of those data. They are not interested in the end result of the processing. If a data controller uses a data processor to handle confidential information on their behalf, there must be a written contract in place that details the responsibilities of each party and the measures in place to protect the data and the rights of the individual under GDPR. Most patient data are collected by hospitals acting as the *data controller* and are used only for the purposes of healthcare. For research purposes, some specified data, with appropriate consent, may be analysed for research by a specialist data analysis organisation, contracted by the NHS. This organisation would be a *data processor*.

The 1997 **Caldicott Review** identified six principles that NHS organisations must adhere to when handling confidential, patient-identifiable information.[4] A seventh was added in 2013 and the eighth in 2020 following further reviews[5,6] (**Figure 16.2**). Every NHS or private sector organisation providing publicly funded healthcare must appoint a **Caldicott guardian**, who is responsible for ensuring that the principles are adhered to.

DATA ACCESS

Access to confidential patient information must be restricted to staff who have a legitimate business or 'patient care' need. Access should be determined by the **information asset owner** (the person responsible for making decisions about information management); this might be the service manager or clinical lead. Information and systems managed by these departments should be subject to an **access control policy**, which

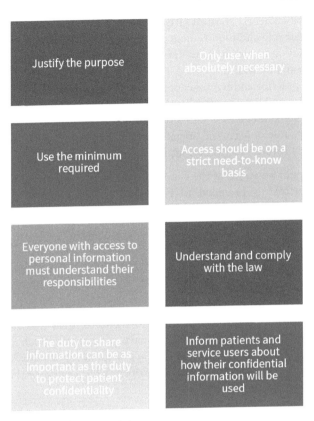

Figure 16.2 The Caldicott principles.

will describe who is able to access the data on these systems and the measures in place to ensure appropriate management, including where data are accessed remotely. Access to data might be managed in several ways:

- physical restrictions: locked access to hard copy film or case note stores;
- individual user logins and passwords; limits to the use of generic logins.
- access privileges/permissions to determine the level of access to data or functionality to the user;

- role-based access controls (RBACs) assigned to the individual based on their role and requirement for types of information;
- policies and procedures to determine how information can be used, when and by whom;
- good practice and housekeeping such as clear-desk/clear-screen policies and logging off when leaving the device;
- management of access for staff who move between departments, change role or leave the organisation;
- strictly limited access periods for agency staff.

Staff should be aware of the conditions and expectations under which system access is provided to them and the consequences of non-compliance. Managing unauthorised access can be challenging as it is impractical to review the access records of every staff member, and even harder to determine if a clinical record was legitimately accessed. Most transactions taking place on an IT system are recorded in the system audit log, meaning that it should be possible to establish what access has taken place and by whom. If a staff member is found to have inappropriately accessed patient information, this is likely to be a breach of the terms of their employment contract and should be managed according to local disciplinary procedures. Such incidents should be reported on the organisation's incident reporting system and may require the Information Commissioner's Office and/or the patient to be informed of the breach.

INFORMATION GOVERNANCE AND ACCOUNTABILITY

Accountability is one of the data protection principles, requiring organisations to take responsibility for compliance with GDPR and to provide evidence to that effect. This may be achieved through ensuring appropriate measures, such as policies, documentation or responsible individuals, are in place to demonstrate compliance. Whenever the processing of personal information is likely to result in a high risk to the rights of the patient, and when introducing new processes or systems, a **data protection impact assessment** (DPIA) must be completed. This is similar to a risk assessment and describes how data are processed and what the data protection risks are. It should provide details of the following:

- how data will be collected, used, stored and deleted;
- where the data will be located/hosted (geographically);
- how the data will be accessed;
- how long the data will be retained;
- what the data flow will look like;
- what governance and contractual arrangements are in place;
- how the rights of data subjects (identifiable individuals about which information is kept) will be upheld;
- risks to data security and to individuals;
- how the risks will be mitigated.

In addition, where arrangements with other organisations or suppliers include the sharing or use of data, there must be a **data-sharing agreement** (DSA) in place. This is a document that defines, in detail, the purpose, processes, standards and responsibilities of data sharing between data controllers. It provides more operational detail than the DPIA, describing the purpose of sharing, what data will be shared and with whom. It sets out the roles and responsibilities of those involved in sharing the data and describes how an individual's rights will be maintained. The organisation must also be registered with the **Information Commissioner's Office** (ICO), an independent organisation set up to regulate data protection laws in the UK, investigate breaches and complaints and issue penalties for infringement where appropriate. If contracts with suppliers include the sharing or use of data, confirmation that the organisation is registered with the ICO may be required.

All personal data breaches should be reported via the organisation's incident reporting system in line with the incident reporting policy. A personal data breach is defined in the GDPR as:

> *a breach of security leading to the accidental or unlawful destruction, loss, alteration, unauthorised disclosure of, or access to, personal data transmitted, stored or otherwise processed.*

An example of this is sending a patient letter to the wrong address. Breaches may also need to be reported to the ICO and to the individuals affected, under the advice of the information governance (IG) team. This team oversees the IG agenda and comprises the:

- **Caldicott guardian:** Responsible for protecting the confidentiality of personal health and care information and making sure it is used accordance with the eight Caldicott principles. This role will usually be held by a very senior member of the organisation, for example the medical director.
- **Data protection officer (DPO):** Responsible for monitoring compliance with GDPR and data protection regulations.
- **Senior information risk owner (SIRO):** An executive director or senior board member responsible for ensuring that information risks are appropriately managed.
- **IG or data security and protection lead:** Accountable for co-ordination and management of the IG programme.

To demonstrate good IG, the organisation must use the **Data Security and Protection Toolkit** (DSPT).[7] This allows organisations to assess their performance against the National Data Guardian's 10 data security standards (**Figure 16.3**), which focus on ensuring staff are able to handle information according to the Caldicott principles, ensuring organisations proactively prevent data security breaches and respond appropriately to incidents and near misses, and ensuring that technology is secure and up to date.

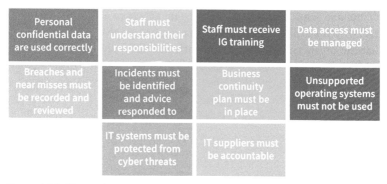

Figure 16.3 National Data Guardian's 10 data security standards.

The **National Data Guardian for Health and Social Care** is a statutory independent role that acts as a champion for patients/the public in ensuring that confidential information is handled correctly.

Information can be shared for the purposes of healthcare in accordance with the strict statutory regulations discussed above. There are also some circumstances where specific information, patient or corporate, may be requested. These are:

1. *Subject access requests.* The GDPR and Data Protection Act 2018 give patients the right to request a copy of information held in their health records. The scope, request and approval processes for the release of specific patient-identifiable information will be documented in organisational policies and must include procedures for assessing, approving and providing information where patients are seeking access to their medical records or where legal firms are requesting access as part of a claim. Copies of records must be provided within 30 days of receipt of the request. There are some exemptions allowing the request to be declined, for example if it is likely to cause serious physical or mental harm to the individual or another person.

2. *Freedom of information (FOI).* The FOI Act[8] allows individuals to request certain information from public bodies, including the NHS. This could include financial, operational and governance information, but does not include personal information. The response to such a request must be within 20 working days of receipt, unless there is a valid reason why this is not possible. FOI requests can be declined in certain circumstances, such as when the request is vexatious, it would be too expensive or time-consuming to respond or it is a repeat request from the same person. In addition, there are some exemptions to the disclosure of certain information, for example if it is commercially sensitive.

RECORDS RETENTION AND DISPOSAL

ISO 15489-1:2016 Information and documentation – Records management[9] defines records as 'Information created, received, and maintained as evidence and as an asset by an organisation or person'.

This includes an individual's health data concerning diagnosis, care or treatment, but also other information such as staff and administrative and research records. Records may be in the form of paper, digital, email/text messages or physical (such as dental moulds). The **NHS Records Management Code of Practice**[10] provides guidance on management, storage and destruction of records, although organisations may also have local record retention policies. The code of practice provides a framework for records management based on established standards and includes guidelines on topics such as legal, professional, organisational and individual responsibilities when managing records. The length of time records should be held will depend on the record type (**Table 16.1**). The code of practice provides guidance on health and care records and on documents/data such as staff and patient surveys, risk and incident logs, duty rosters and financial records.

Once the minimum retention period has been reached and records are no longer required, a process of 'appraisal' should take place to determine what will happen to the records in line with relevant local and national policies or guidelines, with evidence provided of the decision made. There are some specific circumstances where data cannot

Table 16.1 Length of time records should be held.

Record type	Minimum retention period
Adult health records not covered by any other section in this schedule including X-rays and scans	8 years
Children's records	Until 25th birthday (26th if the patient was 17 when treatment ended)
Dental records	15 years
Cancer/oncology records	30 years or 8 years after death
Long-term illness, or illness that may recur records	20 years, or 10 years after death
Staff record	Until 75th birthday
Equipment maintenance logs	11 years
Board and committee meetings	Between 6 and 20 years

be destroyed, for example if they are required for a coroner's inquest. Health record disposal can be complex to manage; manual filing or IT systems may be able to easily identify and destroy records that have reached 8 years of age, but locating and retaining those that include cancer or long-term illness diagnoses, for example, can be far more challenging as there may not be a simple way to flag these within a patient's record. Although most PACS can provide 'image lifecycle' management tools such as automatic rules-based deletion, this requires the ability to identify key data items such as timestamps, clinical codes or patient age. Disease classification, such as SNOMED CT, a structured clinical vocabulary for use in electronic health records,[11] is not always used consistently, or may not have been in place for the records now approaching disposal timescales. A manual review of records to identify those that should be excluded from disposal is generally considered extremely time-consuming and not cost-effective.

Paper records should be destroyed according to ISO 15489-1:2016. For digital records, system-level 'deletion' of digital records may not be sufficient as it can be possible to subsequently recover the data from the hard drive. Deletion of digital records must be audited and should be managed under advice from IT services and system suppliers. Where specialist external companies are used to destroy data, they must have the appropriate ISO accreditation and provide certification or evidence that destruction has taken place.

CHAPTER SUMMARY

- Healthcare informatics is a term used to describe the use of information and technology in the acquisition, processing and analysis of patient data to deliver and improve healthcare.
- 'Data' is defined as 'information, especially facts or numbers, collected to be examined and considered and used to help decision-making'.
- Business intelligence is a term used to describe the use of software that can ingest large volumes of data and provide an overview and interpretation in the form of dashboards, reports and charts.

- AI involves the simulation of human processes by computer systems and is gaining momentum.
- Access to confidential patient information is determined by the information asset owner and should be restricted to staff who have a legitimate business or 'patient care' need.
- In the EU, the legal framework for the protection of an individual's information is the GDPR.
- A Caldicott guardian is responsible for ensuring that NHS organisations adhere to Caldicott principles when handling confidential, patient-identifiable information.
- A DPIA must be completed when introducing new processes or systems and the processing of personal information that may result in a high risk to the rights of the patient.
- Information can be shared for the purposes of healthcare in accordance with the strict statutory regulations and may be requested by individuals through a subject access request or a freedom of information request.
- 'ISO 15489-1:2016 Information and documentation – Records management' defines the length of time records should be held for.

REFERENCES

1. Cambridge Dictionary. Data. Available at https://dictionary.cambridge.org/dictionary/english/data.
2. General Data Protection Regulation (GDPR). Available at https://gdpr.eu/tag/gdpr.
3. Data Protection Act 2018. Available at www.legislation.gov.uk/ukpga/2018/12/contents/enacted.
4. Department of Health and The Caldicott Committee. Report on the Review of Patient-identifiable Information. 1997. Available at https://webarchive.nationalarchives.gov.uk/ukgwa/20130124064947/http://www.dh.gov.uk/prod_consum_dh/groups/dh_digitalassets/@dh/@en/documents/digitalasset/dh_4068404.pdf.
5. Department of Health. Information: To Share or Not to Share – Government Response to the Caldicott Review. 2013. Available at https://assets.publishing.service.gov.uk/media/5a7c4716e5274a2041cf2ebb/9731-2901141-TSO-Caldicott-Government_Response_ACCESSIBLE.PDF.

6. National Data Guardian. The National Data Guardian's Response to the Consultation on the Caldicott Principles and Caldicott Guardians. 2020. Available at https://assets.publishing.service.gov.uk/media/5fcf52a4e90e07562074768a/NDG_CP_and_CG_consultation_response_FINAL_08.12.20.pdf.

7. NHS England. Data Security and Protection Toolkit Assessment Guides. Available at https://digital.nhs.uk/cyber-and-data-security/guidance-and-assurance/data-security-and-protection-toolkit-assessment-guides.

8. Freedom of Information Act 2000. Available at www.legislation.gov.uk/ukpga/2000/36/contents.

9. ISO. ISO 15489-1:2016 Information and Documentation – Records Management. Available at www.iso.org/standard/62542.html.

10. NHS England. Records Management Code of Practice. 2023. Available at https://transform.england.nhs.uk/information-governance/guidance/records-management-code/.

11. NHS England. SNOMED CT. Available at https://digital.nhs.uk/services/terminology-and-classifications/snomed-ct#:~:text=SNOMED%20CT%20is%20a%20structured,clinical%20vocabulary%20readable%20by%20computers.

17. EMERGENCY PREPAREDNESS, RESILIENCE AND RESPONSE

Amanda Martin and Louise Kemp

INTRODUCTION

Emergency preparedness, resilience and response (EPRR) is required within the healthcare sector and is a part of the UK Civil Contingencies Act 2004.[1] Being adequately prepared to deal with any emergency, having the ability to respond instantaneously and having the capability to recover from that emergency is vital in today's health and social care service. There is a national framework that sets out the principles for NHS organisations in responding to emergencies: the **NHS Emergency Preparedness, Resilience and Response Framework**.[2] The key principle is that of oversight and management of any incident that impacts the organisation, but there is also the expectation that each individual organisation will respond in the same way in order to provide some national consistency in responding to such events. Local plans must be developed from these principles, outlining steps to take in a wide range of events that could affect patient care or the health of those living and working in the locality. It is not possible to identify every possible emergency that could occur, but there are commonalities in the way that an organisation would respond and recover, and plans should be aimed at dealing with these.

The local plans must enable the organisation to continue to deliver care if such an event occurs and must clearly address the actions needed. Emergency incidents are categorised in two ways:

DOI: 9781003380078-17

- *Major incidents (MIs)* are those that occur external to the organisation and may require the co-ordinated response of multiple organisations;
- *Critical incidents (CIs) or business continuity incidents (BCIs)* are those that occur internally and, although they may not require a co-ordinated response from other organisations, they may require support in order for business to continue.

MAJOR INCIDENTS

An MI is defined by the Joint Emergency Service Interoperability Programme[3] as 'An event or situation with a range of serious consequences which requires special arrangements to be implemented by one or more emergency responder agency'.

Such events may be:

- an infectious disease outbreak, either a local norovirus infection or a global pandemic;
- adverse weather conditions causing, for example, flooding;
- an MI in the transport sector;
- a terrorist attack;
- a crowd collapse and crush involving many people.

These incidents generally impact large numbers of people; however, hospital services may not necessarily be required, depending on the nature of the incident. For example, there are likely to be few casualties caused by flooding, whereas a multiple vehicle collision may result in large numbers of patients requiring hospital care. If the NHS is required to deliver care, then a standardised response level is issued ranging from level 1 (incident can be managed locally within normal service provision) to level 4 (incident requires central co-ordination by NHS England). This is used across all NHS organisations in England, and it is likely that there are similar processes in other nations; it drives the response to the incident.

In incidents involving casualties, the hospital will be informed by the ambulance incident officer and the agreed action plans will be implemented. It is possible that the hospital will be put on '**standby**' due to the lack of full knowledge of the incident and number of casualties involved. In this instance, only a small number of people will be informed. If it is decided that hospital services are not required, then the incident will be stood down; however, if those services are required, then an MI will be **declared**.

The roles of some staff and the service delivered by some locations may alter during an MI response, so it is important to have quick access to '**action cards**' that outline the role and actions of those involved (**Figure 17.1**). There must be one card for each role, but this may include a single person or multiple people. For example, the radiographers may have an action card relating to their role, which will remain unchanged, but the lead emergency nurse practitioner may be required to relocate to an outpatient setting to ensure that care can still be delivered to patients requiring hospital care but not involved in the incident. The outpatient setting then becomes an extension of the Emergency Department (ED).

It is also essential to have a robust 'call-in' process to ensure that enough staff are available, but not too many so that the services cannot continue to be delivered after the incident is stood down. This can be

Major Incident Action Card - Radiographer	Role: The role of the radiographer taking the standby or activate plan call is to prepare the department to receive patients. This will be done by the following actions.
	1. Inform the senior person in charge and the duty radiologist.
	2. Allocate management of patients in the department to a radiographer.
	3. Allocate preparation of equipment to a radiographer.
	4. Attend the METHANE briefing in the control room.
	5. Determine if any more staff need to be called in and follow the call-in procedure if doing this.
	6. Allocate staff to areas dependent on the METHANE report.
	7. Attend the debrief once the incident is stood down.

Figure 17.1 Example of an action card.

as simple as a paper-based telephone number list, but it can be difficult keeping that updated. Software packages are available, such as WhatsApp, and can be used as long as confidential data are not being shared and it is being used to simply alert staff to the need to attend the workplace. It is generally easier to keep electronic staff lists updated.

One of the first actions, after allocating responsibilities, is for the lead practitioner to attend the control room and receive the **METHANE** report. This is a structured way of ensuring that all organisations, staff groups and individuals receive the same information about the event. This report will include the following:

- **Major incident status** – date and time of incident declaration;
- **Exact location** – this will enable an estimate of casualty arrival time;
- **Type of incident** – this will allow an assessment of the type of injuries to expect and the facilities that may need to be made ready;
- **Hazards** – any current or expected hazards will help in understanding types of injuries, but also any contamination factors, for example from a chemical explosion;
- **Access** – safe routes to the incident for emergency responders, but this also enables an estimate of casualty arrival time too, as limited access will result in delays extracting casualties from the scene;
- **Number of casualties** – this knowledge, along with the above information, will help in planning staffing numbers;
- **Emergency services** – indicates which services are on scene.

This information will inform the planning for receipt of patients. This may require plans to be put in place for patients currently waiting within the department. Decisions must be made on a case-by-case basis by a senior practitioner who has the ability to determine the urgency of any outstanding investigations or treatments. It may be possible to relocate staff to deal with urgent but not incident-related examinations, but some patients may have to be asked to return later.

Staffing allocation may differ depending on the time of day, but it must already have been predetermined how many staff will be needed as a minimum. If the incident is out of hours and staff need to be called to site, then consider the skill mix required based on information from the METHANE report. As tempting as it may be to call in a number of staff for support, consider the staffing needs for the following day. The incident may not be over and rotation of staff in an extended incident is essential to minimise exhaustion, both mental and physical.

Resources must be made available at appropriate locations, for example moving mobile radiography machines into the ED and theatre. Most of this can be done before casualties start to arrive, although it must be recognised that casualties with minor injuries may arrive in their own transportation. This 'upside-down triage' gives time to execute plans before those patients with more significant injuries arrive.

Casualties are categorised as follows:

- P1 – those who need immediate treatment for life-threatening or life-changing injuries;
- P2 – those who need intervention within 6 hours;
- P3 – those who do need treatment, but not immediately or within the next 6 hours.

Patients can transition between these categories, for example if an apparent non-life-threatening injury deteriorates.

Each casualty will have a **unique identifier** (ID), usually a number, which is recorded on all documentation instead of the patient demographics. This unique ID will remain with the patient until they are discharged from ED or admitted to a ward. This may cause challenges if they return for further imaging once admitted, as it may not be immediately identifiable that the patient, who now attends under their own name, has already had imaging. Increased vigilance is needed to ensure that patients are not unduly over-irradiated; local procedures must outline steps to be taken to minimise this risk.

It is essential that training in response to an MI takes place so that staff can test their knowledge about the procedure in relation to their role. This will increase awareness and reduce stress should they be involved in an actual incident and is a requirement of the **Civil Contingencies Act** (2004).[1] There are three types of training exercises,[4] with the easiest and quickest being discussion-based. Staff can talk about the existing plan with somebody who is able to answer any questions that might arise. This is generally profession- or role-specific and should take place every 6 months. A table-top exercise is a simulation of an MI using a real-life scenario and involving a wide range of teams. The scenario is acted out as it would happen, but usually at a much faster pace so that all inputs to the scenario can be assessed. This is generally an annual exercise. A live exercise will be scenario-based, but occurs in the specific locations and at the expected timescale of the incident. Such an exercise puts immense pressure on service delivery, but should be carried out every 3 years.

CRITICAL AND BUSINESS CONTINUITY INCIDENTS

CIs and BCIs affect a single organisation and are declared depending on the impact of the incident.

- A **critical incident** is declared when the organisation cannot deliver critical services.
- A **business continuity incident** may be declared if the service delivery drops below an acceptable level, but the service can still be delivered.

Categorisation of the incident may differ between departments within an organisation. For example, a loss of water supply in one department may be catastrophic, leading to service suspension and declaration of a CI, whereas, in another department, it may simply slow down processes, with the declaration of a BCI. The organisation as a whole would declare a CI if a critical service cannot be delivered. While an organisation-wide incident may impact services differently, there may be an incident that is department-specific. For example, in a radiotherapy department, treatment can be paralysed if the record-and-verify system fails, as this is required to deliver all radiotherapy treatment plans.

The **ISO 22301:2019** is the international standard for implementation of a business continuity management system.[5] Each department must have a business continuity plan, which should include individualised plans to address all possible incidents that may impact their ability to deliver services. The plans should include actions that are defined by the impact on the service. The plans are developed by first identifying the risk and than creating action plans to be implemented should the incident occur.[5] The aim is to ensure service continuity.

There are many elements to a medical imaging or radiotherapy service, and some are not critical to service delivery; therefore, to carry out a risk assessment, it is essential to understand the impact that an incident may have on that service. When considering impacts, it is important to consider not only the delivery of the service, but also the financial impact on the organisation. The following are some points to consider in an incident that affects the department where there is a single point of failure.

1. *Service outcome.* What other departments may be affected if the medical imaging or radiotherapy service can no longer operate to its full capacity? Is this likely to affect the service that other departments can deliver too? Medical imaging affects most services across the hospital, but some may be able to carry on with their normal service, while others may have to consider their ability to operate as normal. This will depend on the type of incident.
2. *Clinical service impact.* What is the impact on the patients affected? Is this incident likely to impact clinical service delivery? It is likely that any incident affecting the medical imaging or radiotherapy service will have an immediate clinical impact, as it is often needed for urgent diagnosis/treatment of critically ill or injured patients. The Royal College of Radiologists has published a document providing guidance on managing unscheduled gaps in radiotherapy treatment for different tumour types.[6] This includes the impact of the duration and the timing of the interruption. Evidence-based categorisation of patients according to their tumour type and treatment intent supports departments to prioritise patients according to the need to manage interruptions.
3. *Business service impact.* This will depend on the extent of the incident. There may be loss of income if patients have to go elsewhere, with the additional expenditure of paying for that alternative service. In addition, the reputation of the organisation may suffer if there are increased patient waits. It is prudent to have plans in place for an alternative service provider to immediately step in if the service fails.

For any incident, the cause must be determined. If it is a local problem that does not impact all areas delivering diagnostic or treatment services, then it may be possible to relocate patients, depending on patient condition and their reason for attendance. This may not be possible if there has been an organisation-wide incident; action cards must indicate the steps to take in such an event. In a radiotherapy setting, identification of the causes of unscheduled treatment interruptions is essential and departments must include procedures in their quality system documents to prevent or minimise the effect of a delay in any radiotherapy treatment.

Action cards will be extremely beneficial for staff to reference in a CI or a BCI. This will be a stressful time and decisions can be impaired. Action cards will focus the mind on those steps that need to be taken to ensure that safe services can still be delivered.

PACS AND IT BUSINESS CONTINUITY

Information technology (IT) business continuity planning can be complex to describe due to the number of variables involved. **Downtime procedures** will be dependent on which system(s) have failed, what system integrations are in place, the degree of paperless working in operation, whether the system has failed in or out of hours, whether the failure is planned or unplanned and whether it is expected to be a short- or long-term failure.

Digital systems are embedded in imaging department workflows, often relying on a number of integrated systems and data flows, from the initial referral to sharing the completed report and supporting all of the steps in between. At the very least, an imaging examination is likely to depend on the use of a radiology information system (RIS), a picture archiving and communication system (PACS) and a patient administration system (PAS); it may often also involve electronic patient records (EPRs), electronic requests/results, bed or Emergency Department management or other specialty/sub-specialty systems. These, of course, will also rely on the hospital network to provide access.

Organisational-level IT and informatics business continuity plans should define actions in the event of a loss of shared systems and networks; however, it is essential to provide local, specialty-specific guidance on how this might affect imaging workflows and what the response should be. The **business continuity plan** should act as a point of reference to describe what actions should be taken to maintain the maximum possible levels of service. A local business continuity approach should align with organisation-level procedures. Paper copies should be readily available in case of loss of access to the network or the intranet.

System Downtime Processes

Fortunately, major prolonged system failures are rare; however, it is important to prepare in advance, as they can be disastrous for service delivery. An effective business continuity plan should be able to provide guidance on every step in the workflow and how digital processes will be replaced during downtime. Where there are significant gaps in service continuity that might affect patient safety, consider adding these to the risk register along with an appropriate action plan. A business continuity plan should describe the business continuity approach so that it can be understood and acted upon by a non-'IT or system expert', such as a radiographer or senior manager on call. That does not mean that technical work will be carried out by them or that they need to understand the technical architecture, but they will need to know what steps to take if an incident takes place and they will need to understand the possible implications of a loss of systems.

Consider the following questions, and whether they can be answered as part of the business continuity plans for different scenarios.

- Referrals
  - How will existing electronic referrals be viewed?
  - How will requests be made if electronic requesting is unavailable?
  - Where are the paper request forms kept? What happens if they run out?

- Booking and appointments
  - How will patients be entered into systems (if hospital IDs are not available)?
  - How will temporary IDs be allocated?

- Imaging examinations
    - Is there a reciprocal agreement with a local organisation to enable urgent examinations to be conducted, should there be a system failure that prevents imaging taking place?
    - How will booked appointments be seen? How will staff know who is attending for what and what the clinical indications are (for electronic referrals) and what the protocol is?
    - How will patients be entered on modalities if there are no worklists and/or if hospital IDs are not available?
    - What happens to the images if they cannot be sent to a PACS? How many examinations can the modality hold, what happens if the modality storage fills up, can images be burned to CD/DVD?
    - Where will radiographers record the post-processing details?
    - Where should the paperwork be kept?
- Reporting
    - Will everything be reported – how will reporting be prioritised?
    - Where will images be reported from? Are they accessible from PACS workstations or will they need to have a provisional review from the modality?
    - How will reports be dictated/transcribed?
    - How will reporters know what is waiting to be reported?
    - How will we know if reports have been handwritten in notes and what the report said?
- Image and report viewing
    - How will users access and view new (during downtime) and historical (pre-downtime) images and reports?
    - How will staff log in to temporary or business continuity systems?
    - How should users search for patients? Can they still use hospital IDs or NHS numbers?
    - How can images and reports be shared with other external organisations?
    - How will mobile or urgent imaging be viewed by the referrer?

It may be useful to provide an IT business continuity folder containing all the items that might be needed in such an event, for example laminated action cards, pre-printed provisional report stickers, paper request cards and a temporary patient log; this will help when cross-checking that requests/images/reports have been uploaded after the event.

Fault Reporting

During normal working hours, the imaging informatics/PACS or IT team is likely to be the first point of contact for dealing with system failures. Out of hours, it is important to support the staff and operational requirements to maintain the service to the maximum capabilities, reducing delays to clinicians and risks to patients.

Guidance is needed for out-of-hours working to clarify the following.

- Will radiographers contact the on-call IT team or the supplier directly?
- When and how to contact the PACS manager or imaging informatics team.
- What are the relevant supplier or help-desk contact numbers/email addresses?
- Are faults logged online? How is this accessed? Do urgent faults need to be followed up with a phone call?
- What serial numbers or system IDs might need to be quoted?
- What constitutes an urgent fault? What should be done about non-urgent faults?
- Escalation pathways.
- Expected response times and service-level agreements.
- Severity descriptors.
- Who needs to be informed?
- What additional information might the on-call IT team need to support the fault resolution and business continuity?

Action Cards

Action cards are a highly effective tool for describing different scenarios and the action required (**Figure 17.2**). They should be written from the perspective of the service (staff in imaging department) and the users (in this scenario, this will be the clinicians and other clinical staff) and should include all the information necessary to identify and manage the downtime.

Communication

Good communication is an essential part of business continuity, enabling service users to plan and adapt to the incident. Inform service users of the failure, particularly those who rely heavily on the service, and provide details of relevant downtime procedures, such as how to make referrals, view images and/or access imaging reports. Depending on the circumstances, it may be helpful to inform senior leaders, such as patient flow co-ordinators and divisional management. They will be able to assist in cascading the impact of the incident to relevant teams. It is useful to have a pre-written email template available to circulate at short notice, assuming network functions such as email communications are available. Once systems are available again, this should be communicated in the same way.

Planned Downtime

Planned downtime, for example due to system upgrades, is often arranged out of hours, although more lengthy downtimes may tip over into standard working hours. It allows wards and departments to plan ahead according to the duration and type of the downtime. It may be prudent to consider reducing planned lists (both in radiology and

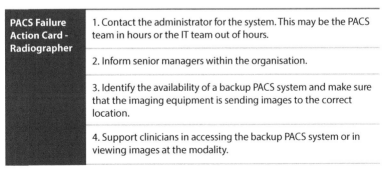

PACS Failure Action Card - Radiographer	1. Contact the administrator for the system. This may be the PACS team in hours or the IT team out of hours.
	2. Inform senior managers within the organisation.
	3. Identify the availability of a backup PACS system and make sure that the imaging equipment is sending images to the correct location.
	4. Support clinicians in accessing the backup PACS system or in viewing images at the modality.

Figure 17.2 Example of a PACS failure action card.

in outpatient clinics) or increasing staffing to support the additional workload linked to manual entry and paper-based systems and the subsequent post-downtime measures.

Most radiotherapy record-and-verify systems will receive an annual update that will require a complete system shutdown. This is usually done at weekends and planned many months in advance. Arrangements must be made and agreed with a neighbouring radiotherapy centre to ensure emergency treatments can continue to be delivered, for example radiotherapy for metastatic spinal cord compression. Thorough plans, including transportation of the patient and sharing of radiology images and patient records, must all be developed, tested and confirmed well in advance.

Post-downtime Procedures

Once systems are back in operation, some work will need to be done to ensure that all patient records are checked and complete. This may include backloading referrals and post-processing data and sending images to PACS. Plans should include who is responsible and what checks should take place to ensure that all of the record is complete.

Following downtime of a radiotherapy record-and-verify system, thorough testing must be carried out to ensure that the system is fully operational in advance of the next clinical day.

Learning from Downtime Incidents

Ideally, business continuity processes should be tested before they are needed to make sure the procedures work as expected – a real system downtime incident is not the best time to find out that something is missing or doesn't work as planned. Following a test or actual incident, there should be a debrief and review of the plan to assess whether it can be updated or improved, and resources such as printed plans of paper request cards should be replaced or reordered as needed.

CHAPTER SUMMARY

- Being adequately prepared to deal with any emergency, having the ability to respond instantaneously and having the capability to recover from that emergency is vital in today's health and social care service.
- Local plans must be in place to enable an organisation to continue to deliver care if an incident takes place.
- Major incidents are those that occur external to the organisation and may require the co-ordinated response of multiple organisations.
- Critical incidents or business continuity incidents are those that occur internally and, although they may not require a co-ordinated response from other organisations, they may require support in order for business to continue.
- A critical incident is declared when the organisation cannot deliver critical services.
- A business continuity incident may be declared if the service delivery drops below an acceptable level, but the service can still be delivered.
- IT business continuity planning can be complex due to the number of systems used.
- Downtime procedures must be in place.
- Action cards outline the role and actions of those involved in responding to an incident.

REFERENCES

1. Civil Contingencies Act 2004. Available at www.legislation.gov.uk/ukpga/2004/36/contents.
2. NHS England. NHS Emergency Preparedness, Resilience and Response Framework. 2022. Available at www.england.nhs.uk/publication/nhs-emergency-preparedness-resilience-and-response-framework/.
3. Joint Emergency Service Interoperability Programme (JESIP). Major Incident. Available at www.jesip.org.uk/webapp/major.html.

4.   Gov.uk. Emergency Planning and Preparedness: Exercises and Training. 2013. Available at www.gov.uk/guidance/emergency-planning-and-preparedness-exercises-and-training.

5.   ISO. ISO 22301:2019 Security and Resilience – Business Continuity Management Systems – Requirements. Available at www.iso.org/standard/75106.html.

6.   Royal College of Radiologists. Timely Delivery of Radical Radiotherapy: Guidelines for the Management of Unscheduled Treatment Interruptions. Fourth edition. 2019. Available at www.rcr.ac.uk/our-services/all-our-publications/clinical-oncology-publications/timely-delivery-of-radical-radiotherapy-guidelines-for-the-management-of-unscheduled-treatment-interruptions-fourth-edition/.

INDEX

Note: Page numbers in *italics* refer to figures.

*For Product Safety Concerns and Information please contact
our EU representative GPSR@taylorandfrancis.com Taylor & Francis
Verlag GmbH, Kaufingerstraße 24, 80331 München, Germany*

T - #0211 - 160425 - C296 - 198/129/14 - PB - 9781032436159 - Gloss Lamination